Eat Sweat Play

Anna Kessel is a sports writer for the *Guardian* and the *Observer*. She is also the co-founder and chair of Women in Football.

ANNA KESSEL

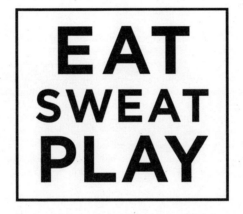

How Sport Can Change Our Lives

MACMILLAN

First published 2016 by Macmillan
an imprint of Pan Macmillan
20 New Wharf Road, London N1 9RR
Associated companies throughout the world
www.panmacmillan.com

ISBN 978-1-5098-0809-0

1 3 5 7 9 8 6 4 2

A CIP catalogue record for this book is available from the British Library.

Printed and bound by CPI Group (UK) Ltd, Croydon, CR0 4YY

Visit **www.panmacmillan.com** to read more about all our books
and to buy them. You will also find features, author interviews and
news of any author events, and you can sign up for e-newsletters
so that you're always first to hear about our new releases.

For Leon, Ella and Malaika

Contents

Introduction

I didn't think I could write a book about women and sport. I don't play sport, I bunked PE my whole school life, and if a ball comes anywhere near my face I blink. I get nervous walking past a game of football in case I have to kick the ball back to someone, and spectacularly fail. Which is kind of a career hazard considering I've been a sports journalist for the last twelve years.

So when the idea was first suggested to me I said no. Short of a chronic case of impostor syndrome, I couldn't imagine preaching to a converted audience of hardcore sports lovers. What would be the point? These women are already out there doing their thing. The issue is that there are all too few of them. The majority of the female population doesn't engage in sport, either playing it, or watching it. Why is that?

The more I thought about it, the more I thought about the contradictions. Most of my female friends don't call themselves sports fans, but they get excited about watching Wimbledon, or the World Cup or the Olympics. They might not exercise regularly, but they've probably done a 10km, or played badminton or table tennis. They just didn't necessarily like PE, or can't remember who won the FA Cup. And the women who *are* crazy about sport aren't getting an easy time of it because society casually dubs them unfeminine, or rubbish at it, or lesser sports fans than men. So that as women, whether we love sport or loathe it, we are constantly being defined as incompatible with it. Alien. Odd. Other.

For men, sport and exercise are all part of the same active spectrum, but for women they are presented as two very distinct things. Exercise, with its approved end-goal of delivering you a better body, is revered for twenty-first-century women. From the launch of Net-A-Sporter, serving up sports clothing for fashionistas, to the introduction of #plankie and #fitspo for the Instagram generation, exercise for women has gone mainstream. Where once celebrities were forced to sneak out of the back door of a gym, red-faced, now the likes of Victoria Beckham and Ellie Goulding proudly head out on four-mile runs or for boxing sessions in the park. What was formerly known as the 'sweat patch of shame' is now triumphantly circled in gossip magazines, a mark to be revered.

But sport for women is seen as distinct from all this activity. Sweating from sporting exertion is not seen as beautiful. Its *raison d'être* strays too far from appearance. And that's precisely why sport is so important for women. It's a rare moment in our lives, when the emphasis is on playing, being in the now. It's also about determination and grit, not losing a few pounds or looking great, but absolutely wiping the floor with your opponents. It's about winning, showing aggression, being competitive, openly rejoicing and being proud in doing all of these things. It's also about fun. And, when we really think hard about it, women are not encouraged to have fun very often. Unless you buy into advertising-speak about tampons, curling your hair and shopping for a kitchen.

So why *is* sport consistently defined as male territory? Who decides that TV cameras, replicating the male gaze, should habitually seek out the most beautiful women in the crowd? When will women ever flock to watch football, rugby and boxing in their millions? Or turn up to the park with friends for a Sunday morning kickabout? How long do we have to wait to see the first multimillionaire female footballer or basketball player? And what is it really like to be an elite female athlete? Never mind training regimes, what happens if you reach the Wimbledon final and you're on your period? In fact, what even is the deal with exercise and periods? Has anyone researched this stuff? Who are the scientists looking at how boobs respond to exercise, whether female orgasms help or hinder women from winning trophies, and whether you can run off your PMT? Have we even figured out what to call our bodies? When I had to decide on a word for vagina to tell my daughter, I was horrified to discover that other mums were proposing a range of bizarre and confusing terms including moomoo, nunnie, front bottom, bits, flower and twinkle. No wonder grown women – and men – still struggle with how to speak about the female anatomy.

The absence of answers to so many of these questions says it all. Let's face it, society still just isn't that comfortable with real women's bodies, particularly not the sporty and female ones. While we idolize British heptathlete Jessica Ennis-Hill, an Olympic goddess with a six-pack is sadly still not viewed as a role model for many women and young girls. And that is because women are still being sold the myth that sport compromises your femininity (unless you're doing it in your knickers, Lingerie Football League). Because, as society keeps telling us, women are *married to* sports stars – not sports stars in their own right.

Hallelujah, then, that slowly – ever so slowly – a change has come upon us. From Michelle Obama slam-dunking LeBron James at the White House and opening the conversation about physical activity, to baseball's overnight household name Mo'ne Davis who kicked ass in 2014, beating the boys in the Little League World Series, England's women's rugby team winning the World Cup (forcing some of the most conservative sports editors in Fleet Street to put their photo on the front page), England's women footballers winning over a nation, and the steady trickle of women's-interest magazines finally beginning to treat sport as a serious topic to engage their readers.

Still, on pitching this book to publishers I worried that they wouldn't get it. The whole premise of the idea seemed impossibly contradictory: I wanted to appeal to women who didn't connect to sport, who didn't buy sports books, and I wanted to do it with a book about sport. The words of the *Cosmo Body* editor who said her readers were 'scared' of the word sport rang loud in my ears. Surely, this project was flawed.

Amazingly, Macmillan didn't think so. And their leap of faith paid off as Sport England's massive 'This Girl Can' campaign launched in January 2015, speaking to exactly that disenfranchised audience of women that I wanted to reach. When I first watched that advert, Missy Elliott's 'Get Ur Freak On' blaring over a powerful series of moving images, I cried. Because the film showed a realness that is scarily absent from our everyday consumption of female imagery. We saw a range of body types, ethnicities, ages, activities. Best of all, we saw them sweating, smiling, out of breath, with messed-up hair, not concerned about how they looked. We saw them in what would normally be described as varying states of imperfection, and yet here they were *enjoying themselves*. I know not everyone loves the campaign; some critics feel it is not diverse enough, or that 'girl' is an inappropriate term for 'female'. I do not dismiss their concerns, but for me the campaign was a revelation. And best of all, it was cool, not patronizing. Gone were the preachy messages about health and well-being. This Girl Can was about fun and friendship. The fact that they'd chosen Missy to deliver the soundtrack said it all. Missy Elliott, a powerful and all-too-rare female figure in a music industry consumed by misogyny. For my generation of women Missy is all about embracing body image ('Love my guts, so fuck a tummy tuck'), supporting other female artists and female empowerment. She raps about cunnilingus and turning herself on, and in her videos she celebrates the female body without objectifying or denigrating it. And, mostly, she does it all in a tracksuit.

Cue Lena Dunham, Golden Globe award-winning writer, director and star of the hit US TV series *Girls*, who recently noted that 'It ain't about the ass, it's about the brain.' It's got to be *the* slogan for women and girls in the twenty-first century. Lena was talking about running, which she says helped her tackle anxiety in a way that sixteen years of medication never managed to. But she doesn't equate exercise with losing weight, or being healthy, or any of that boring, polarized, feel-bad stuff. Instead she talks about the revelation of being able to run down the street when you're late, actually using your body for its original intended purpose.

There is a realness about Lena that is absent from the mainstream media. She doesn't buy into the bullshit line about all larger women being curvy. She says she has a big body with small breasts and an arse that wouldn't be serenaded in music videos. It's a body shape that we don't acknowledge or celebrate in our culture. And yet it is one that we see every day in the women around us, in ourselves. She rails against women's bodies being politicized and 'policed'. 'We can no longer keep women from owning property. We can no longer keep women from voting. But we will find a way to police and repress powerful women and let them know that they do not matter to us and that they are not in control of their own destiny ... And then women join in because that's what they're being taught from the time they're born. They don't even recognize that they're agents of their own oppression. Not to sound too much like I'm, like, Andrea Dworkin-ing out on you ...'[1]

This book, too, is about challenging the status quo. Society's stereotypes tell us that women don't like sport, but when we really think about it that doesn't make any sense. Isn't the fundamental principle of being physically active something that comes naturally to us from the moment we begin to walk? Don't we all remember our childhoods, running down a hill so fast it made us laugh until we couldn't breathe? Daring ourselves to climb a tree, to do our first cartwheel, our first handstand? What happened to us? When did we change? When did we lose our sense of fun, our sense of play? Sport is just playing, after all. And exercise is just moving our bodies, not hard penance.

Why does any of this matter? Because, as Nelson Mandela

famously put it, 'Sport has the power to change the world.' In some cases, quite literally. Around the globe, projects involving sport are changing women's lives right now. Whether that's teaching women in southern India to swim – following the Asian tsunami of 2004 in which up to four times as many women died as men – or using sport as the vehicle for change by encouraging female leadership skills, raising awareness of HIV/AIDS, offering alternative pathways to prostitution and tackling domestic violence. Why sport? Because it teaches women to take ownership of their bodies, it gives them physical strength, and it gifts them status and new-found respect in cultures where sport is seen as an activity solely for men.

It's time for women the world over to reconnect with our bodies. To reclaim them from a life of obsessing about thigh gaps and bingo wings. To remember that our bodies are there to have fun with, to enjoy. And to make sure that we learn these lessons before it is too late, before we are physically infirm and looking back over our lives wishing we'd tried wild swimming, or netball, or trampolining, wondering what it might have been like to body slam someone on a rugby pitch, or learn how to throw a real punch. What are we waiting for? The daring amongst us, the heroes and rebels, have been bucking the trend and enjoying sport for millennia. From the women of Ancient Greece running barefoot races and medieval nuns playing cricket, to the Tudor women who watched tennis and loved a round of golf. In our own era some of the highest-profile women in the world have fallen in love with sport – from Rihanna to J. K. Rowling and Mary Berry.

This book is about encouraging women and girls to reclaim sport on their own terms. It is not a lecture about health, but rather an invitation to discover the fun and fulfilment in physical activity, and everything that it brings – from better emotional stability to better relationships. It's not about telling women who to be, or what to do; Lord knows we have enough of that in our lives already. And it's not about having a go at men, many of whom would heartily welcome a new de-gendered approach to sport and exercise.

But it *is* about urging us to rethink the spaces that we close off from ourselves. One of the most profound interviews I conducted for this book was with a mother of two children who had taken up boxing, despite hating the sport, and found herself retraining as an archaeologist after years in a 'sensible' desk job. Doing sport literally changed her life. Because, she reasoned, if she could work up the guts to punch someone she could actually do anything. In sport she found a space to escape the pressures and expectations placed upon us as women, from looking perfect to juggling careers and motherhood. Best of all, she found an activity that she fell in love with.

After all, whether we like it or not, sport is everywhere. In our school sports lessons, dominating our TV schedules ('What? *EastEnders* is delayed *again*?'); it's there in our relationships, in our workplace, in the conversations of the world's biggest power-brokers, and it's there dictating our futures. So why don't we start *owning* it? Sport for women and girls is now understood to be so monumentally important and life-changing that even the United Nations have suggested it will play a leading role in the journey to equal rights for women and girls this century. First, though, we've got to get on the scoresheet.

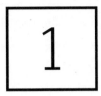

How to bunk a PE lesson: a rough guide

Of all the school sports horrors – bench netball, hockey and cross-country – swimming was the absolute abomination. Sitting on the side of a public pool, arms over your head, perched and ready to practise a seated dive. From that position all you could see was your thighs. I remember staring at mine, unhappy at the view. Pale skin encasing pale adolescent flab spread across the cracked swimming-pool tiles. I was one of the unlucky ones whose thighs merged unstoppably into one enormous, shapeless mass, riddled with blue veins. They hadn't invented the term 'thigh gap' then, but I didn't need anyone to tell me I didn't have one. Bugger the diving technique, all I could think about was how horrible my legs looked.

The swimming itself was awful, of course. Gulps of heavily chlorinated pissed-in water, red stinging eyes, splashing, flailing and thirty minutes later we were out again, scrambling for our towels, struggling with sticky skin catching on our clothes while our PE teachers yelled at us to hurry up. Piling back onto the school bus, we yanked brushes through dripping-wet hair, and shifted uncomfortably as drops pooled on the back of our necks, dampening our clothes. Swimming was humiliating. As far as I could tell, that was the purpose of it.

And so we bunked PE. Come winter, come summer, by Year 9 we were regular absentees. And proud. For a while we tried an intermediary measure – forging a parent's note. *Dear Ms R, Anna is suffering with a heavy cold today and won't be able to take part in PE. Yours sincerely, Inge Kessel.* I wrote it in my best pen, using my left hand so that it didn't look like my own handwriting. But as time passed we grew shameless and emboldened, and soon began strolling out of the school gates with only a quick rearward glance, before legging it out and away to freedom. Perched on a low wall by some public tennis courts (the irony), my friends smoked and we all revelled in the delight of a free period.

Up and down the country the same anti-PE ritual was taking place for teenage girls. My friend Samantha recalls PE at her secondary school in Bournemouth. She and her friends didn't bunk, they just lit up a bong. Crowding together in a toilet at the leisure centre where the school had their swimming lessons, Sam and her mates got a water pipe going with a lump of hash, in the days before smoke alarms were mandatory in every public space. 'We'd get in the pool, stoned out of our heads, going, "The water's like jelly, man. This is *sooo* cool!" Instead of swimming lengths, we'd walk all the way along to the deep end, arms out in breaststroke style, pretending to swim. We thought we were so clever, fooling the teacher. She must have noticed, stood up there on the side, looking down over the water. She obviously just didn't give a shit.'

PE's saving grace was dance. Ms Farley was my hero. Blonde bob, grey leggings, spaghetti-strap tops, and a warm-up routine to Whitney Houston's version of 'I'm Every Woman' that sent shivers down my spine. It was my favourite part of the class, dancing to that song. I don't know why, but it still gets me now. I wouldn't have bunked dance if you'd paid me.

Dance aside, PE was all too often focused on de-feminizing. The message rang out loud and clear: being female was incompatible with being sporty. Strap your boobs down, tie your hair back, ignore your monthly cycles and get on with it. Heaven help the girls who said they couldn't go swimming because they were on their periods. Our head of PE would mock them loudly, and then reach for the nasty-looking tampons in a box in the PE cupboard. But what thirteen-year-old wants to struggle with a PE-store-cupboard tampon, when it's bad enough just getting your head around having a period in the first place? Being a woman, it seemed, just wasn't sporty.

Maybe that's why Flo-Jo – the American sprinter, Florence Griffith Joyner – was so inspirational when I was growing up. Flo-Jo was a double world record holder, world and Olympic champion, but most importantly of all – for me as a young girl – she was an aspirational female sporting icon. With long flowing hair reaching all the way down her back, bright-red lipstick, big jewellery, painted nails and iconic one-legged sprint suits, Flo-Jo wasn't just ripping up the track; she was cool, and redefining what a female sporting hero looked like. I watched her on TV with my brother, Stef, and his American dad, Frankie. Flo-Jo was my real-life She-Ra, Princess of the Universe – glamorous twin sister of 1980s cartoon superhero He-Man. Powerful and strong, She-Ra could throw men, robots and rocks. I loved She-Ra, though looking at her now through adult eyes I admit to being a bit horrified. She had cleavage, for

Christ's sake! And a crotch-skimming miniskirt, and thigh-length high-heeled gold boots!

At the time She-Ra symbolized something rebellious and cool to me, the idea that a strong woman could be sexy. But fast forward a generation and it now feels very outdated. Unfortunately, we haven't quite outgrown this trope. You've only got to google 'sportswomen' to see that one of the first suggested search terms is 'hottest'. Being sporty and sexy is all good and positive in many ways, but in the twenty-first century it's not refreshing enough. It's too often the fundamental criterion for sportswomen to be accepted in the mainstream. Surely we want to get to a point where women can be strong and powerful and *not* sexy. Or only sexy when they feel like it, not as a requirement to getting media coverage or being valued.

When I was growing up girls didn't have posters of sportswomen on their walls. In the 1990s if you wanted a poster on your bedroom wall, the now-defunct chain of shops called Athena pretty much dictated the law. There was a poster for girls: a muscly man stripped to the waist holding a naked baby – just what every young girl yearned for, a child with a hunk. And a poster for boys: the now-iconic image of a woman lifting her tennis skirt to reveal her naked and perfectly pert buttocks. Girls weren't sold sportswomen as inspirational icons, so if you did have a sports star on your bedroom wall it was likely to be a hunky footballer, reproduced in the poster pages of a teenage girls' favourite, *Just Seventeen* magazine (RIP): the likes of Ryan Giggs, Jamie Redknapp or Lee Sharpe. The only exception to this that I ever encountered were gymnasts and horses. Personally I bucked the trend and chose comedienne Maureen Lipman for my bedroom wall, the Jewish grandmother I never had.

For my generation there were three sportswomen who stood out: Flo-Jo, Martina Navratilova and Steffi Graf. Navratilova was my mum's favourite. For a woman who never watched sport, and routinely denounced it as nationalist anti-intellectual machismo bullshit, my mum was all over Wimbledon. Navratilova neatly contravened all of my mum's anti-sports arguments because she was *a)* originally from my mum's native Czechoslovakia; *b)* intelligent ('she wore glasses and, anyway, you could just tell'); *c)* wore shorts: therefore a revolutionary feminist. To me, being a bit of a tomboy at the time, any girl or woman who wore shorts when they were widely expected to be wearing skirts was a natural hero. Every afternoon during Wimbledon I would come home and lounge on the sofa for hours with my mum watching tennis and hardly saying a word, except to let the dogs in or out if they scratched at the door. I'm not sure my mum actually knew the rules of the game, certainly she didn't seem aware of the complexities of a great backhand, but together we sat, spellbound by the movement of bodies across courts, and the gentle sounds of an afternoon of tennis.

Then Steffi Graf came along, and started winning everything. She was undoubtedly an awesome player, but to my twelve-year-old self she was a traitor. I just couldn't understand why – when Navratilova had already broken the mould and wore shorts – anyone would take a step backwards and wear a skirt. As far as I was concerned, Steffi was letting us all down.

Their combined sporting legacy lives on in the inspirational sportswomen of today – Serena Williams, and a stable of amazing track stars such as multi gold-medallist sprinter Allyson Felix, the US 400m specialist Sanya Richards-Ross, double

Olympic-champion Jamaican sprinter Shelly-Ann Fraser-Pryce, or Britain's very own Christine Ohuruogu. My current favourite is US middle-distance runner Alysia Montaño. In 2014 she made headlines for running in the national championships while thirty-four weeks pregnant. She was swiftly dubbed an icon, and even a *Daily Mail* columnist had to admit she was inspirational. I loved Alysia from even before then, covering her races while working the circuit as an athletics correspondent. The American runner always stood out for wearing a flower in her hair, and I loved her explanation. 'I think when people look at women in sport, there's always this sort of, "You run like a girl," and it's almost like a negative thing,' she said. 'I think what the heck is that supposed to mean? Why not run like a girl? We have grit and I can wear a flower in my hair. I can represent femininity and I can represent strength at the same time.'

These athletes grew up in the same era as me, and yet they survived the assault of negative messages about women and sport to flourish as elite sportswomen. Thank goodness they did. Many of them still don't receive the recognition they deserve – Shelly-Ann Fraser-Pryce, for example, may be three times world champion and double Olympic champion over 100m, but how many have heard of her achievements versus her compatriot, Usain Bolt? Nevertheless, they are out there, role models for young girls, many of them outspoken on issues of gender pay equality, or, as in Alysia's case, challenging our ideas around motherhood and sporting careers.

It was years later, as a sports journalist, that I actually got to meet Martina Navratilova, interviewing her in the back of a taxi.[2] I was nervous, she was grumpy. It turned out to be the

most surreal interview of my career, with the conversation rang-
ing from breast cancer and US military policy to Lady Gaga, a
mysterious accident with a French cat, and Battersea Dogs'
Home. Halfway through, and clearly bored with my questions,
Navratilova suddenly leaned out of the window and started
chatting to a French bulldog huffing and puffing its way up a
hill in Putney.

'Hey! So cute,' she yelled out to the dog. 'What's his name?'

'Snoopy,' said the dog's – quite frankly – stunned owner.

'Snoopy?' said Navratilova, adopting a baby voice. 'You don't
look like a Snoopy to me. I have a French bulldog and his name
is Spike. Hey Snoopy. Look up here! Oh, he's so cute.' Snoopy's
owner, still struggling to come to terms with the fact that one
of the world's most famous tennis players was talking to her
dog, finally plucked up the courage to ask a question herself.

'Enjoying the tennis, Martina?' she asked.

'Yeah,' she replied airily, and promptly wound up her window
as the traffic moved on.

During my research in preparation for meeting her, I was
horrified to read that tennis crowds had rarely warmed to
Navratilova as a player. That, like Serena Williams, Navratilova
was often described in freakish terms, sneered at for being too
muscular, or too dominant in their sport. 'Serena is so physically
dominating, people are feeling sorry for her opponents,' nodded
Navratilova, reflecting on their similarities from the back of the
taxi. 'They were feeling sorry for mine. I was very strong, I was
very muscular and I played a very aggressive game. But it's
because she is so strong that she wins and she's proud of her
body. She doesn't apologize for it and I like that. She's like,
"Hey, I'm a strong woman and get out of my way." If she was a

guy they'd love it, but they get intimidated by women being that strong. I empathize with that because I definitely went through it. It's tough because you feel like you're fighting [against the crowd] – it's hard enough fighting the opponent. And you do feel it, you know, not getting that love. It's not fair.'

Even today sportswomen must feel like they are fighting against the crowd, against mainstream society, against expectations. Take women's tennis – then, as now, still all too often valued in terms of how sexy the players are. Sexy = popular. Sexy = cash. When a major sports channel advertised the women's tour on UK television in 2014 they ran the slogan, 'Here come the glamour girls.' It seems insane that all these years later, long after Navratilova's heyday, we are still portraying elite sportswomen in this way. 'It is degrading,' agreed Navratilova, 'because they're not talking about them as a person or as an athlete, they're talking about them as a sexual object. I don't like that.'

Beyond Flo-Jo and Navratilova there weren't enough inspirational female icons in the 1980s. Thank goodness, then, for the Saturday night hit entertainment show *Gladiators*. In 1992 the show launched in Britain and it made a huge impression on me. Yes, the women did wear pink crop tops and shorts but the entire cast of female stars were rippling with muscle. This was a revelation. The female Gladiators were *fierce*, even the smiley ones like Jet and Lightning; they wanted to beat their opponent and I loved how seriously they took each event, hounding contestants up The Wall, virtually pulling their arms out of their sockets on Hang Tough, and whacking them with giant cotton buds in Duel.

Jet was the Gladiator who garnered the most attention, the one whose name everyone knew, and the one everyone fancied.

All these years later I was curious to know what it was like being Jet, 'the sexy one', and I resolved to track her down. I didn't expect to find her working at a medical clinic in North Wales, contributing to building pathways in wellness for work with YouTrain, solving the obesity crisis and supporting those with mental health issues. A trained psychotherapist and teacher, Diane mostly lives her life away from the limelight now, and the kids she works with probably have no idea of how famous she once was. For someone so frequently depicted as smiley, sexy, hair-flicky, she surprises me by how serious she is. While the general public saw her grinning and looking glamorous on *Gladiators*, she was in fact only just turning the corner out of a troubled adolescence during which she had suffered bulimia.

'I had body dysmorphia in my early teens,' she says now. 'I hated the fact I was a very muscular female.' Growing up, the other kids at school made fun of her physique. 'They'd say, "Urgh, look at your calves, you're really muscly!" I was very conscious of it. As a child I found it difficult to accept my body shape. At gymnastics I was tall for my age group; I was the shape of a senior by the age of twelve when the other juniors were very underdeveloped. I had that hang-up of being the bigger girl among the junior squad.' She decided she could never make it as a gymnast – or a dancer – because she wasn't skinny enough. And so the bulimia began. 'I remember that feeling of self-hate,' she says quietly, 'and now I think how can I not have liked food? How can I have used food as a weapon? It caused a lot of sadness. As an athlete I would have performed even better, I'm sure, had I eaten properly.'

A chance audition for *Gladiators* ended up changing her life.

'I was twenty-two when *Glads* first hit the TV screens, I remember thinking it was a relief that a bunch of us women were out there in our Lycra sports outfits being strong athletic women, rather than this heroin-chic image of thin women with eating disorders. I was so proud to be one of these very athletic women with backgrounds of bodybuilding, and athletics, or in my case dance and gymnastics. I felt so proud that we were exemplifying women being very tough and strong.' ITV advised Diane to go public with the history of her eating disorders to avoid any leaks coming out in the newspapers. Her confession followed Andrew Morton's infamous book detailing Princess Diana's own struggles with bulimia. Diane says she found the process healing. 'I'd get letters from girls writing into the show saying, "I hear you were bulimic, look at you now, I'd love to be like you," and I thought that's great because I'm very healthy and a normal body weight.

'*Gladiators* changed things for women, it wasn't a place where you could just stand around and look pretty – you would have been beaten all the time. But also it hurt; there were a lot of injuries and I left after four and a half years when I suffered a spinal injury and nearly broke my neck.' But if the female Gladiators were the embodiment of muscle, I say, how did Diane feel about being labelled the sexy one in pretty much every hot list going that decade? 'I genuinely think it was because I was a bit fatter than the others,' she laughs. 'I had boobs and a big bum, whereas my fellow Gladiators were more athletic than me. I used to grin madly when the cameras were on me and it was a nervous grin. I also had a very high win-count and I think the audience liked that. People would say, "Ooh, she's good at those cartwheels!" Yeah, and there was a reason for it, I couldn't bear standing still in front of people looking at my arse. If there was an opportunity for me to do a barani flip and escape the cameras, I'd do it.'

Diane says there was only one occasion on the show when she felt she was forced into being sexy. Nigel Lythgoe, a.k.a. Nasty Nigel, was director of the programme and he decided to line up the female Gladiators for a shot in front of the contestants' prizes – a blue Jeep for the guys, and a red Jeep for the women. Diane rolls her eyes at the memory. 'I mean, come on, guys! And what really got me, and I've never been a diva, I've always been the consummate professional, but they said, "Girls, please go and stand next to the jeeps. Tracksuits off, just stand around the vehicles." I said, "What? You're asking us to drape ourselves over cars, like bloody Pirelli girl calendar models? No, no, no, I'm a Gladiator. I run around the arena, I don't stand and pose next to a car like a glamour model." I wasn't going to stand next to a car with my arse on show. When I was standing on the podium or swinging around in Hang Tough, or scaling The Wall, I was moving and doing my job as an athlete. It was the one and only time I felt objectified by the producers of the show.'

If Gladiators, Flo-Jo, Navratilova and She-Ra were the powerful female icons of my 1980s upbringing, then the Spice Girls were the self-proclaimed 'girl power' role models of the 1990s. I was seventeen by the time the Spice Girls burst into our consciousness with the catchy hit 'Wannabe', and already too old to be inspired by them. In that teenage angst-ridden way I was searching for complex identities, and found their thematically arranged Spice doctrine – each band member limited to displaying a single trait – irritatingly reductive. I had just fallen in love with football as, that same summer, England hosted the European Championships and the nation went football crazy. The idea of Melanie Chisholm being 'the sporty one' because she wore tracksuits was silly to me. It also seemed instantly to confirm that sporty meant the opposite of glamorous, sexy and feminine, because while Chisholm danced around in trackies, her bandmates wore slinky dresses and heels. In response, the mainstream media made it quite clear which of the Spice Girls we should be letching over. As Ali G. cruelly asked in his Comic Relief interview with Posh and Becks, 'If the best footballer goes out with the fittest Spice Girl, does Sporty Spice go out with someone from Scunthorpe United?'

Back then there was a lot of talk about the Spice Girls being a manufactured band, a marketer's dream – it made me wonder if Sporty Spice even liked sport? Wearing tracksuits wasn't proof enough for me, since that's just leisurewear circa 1993. I had to find out. A trip to a posh hotel in central London on a mission to interview Sporty Spice about sport was an experience in itself.[3] For a sports journalist, sports interviews are nothing like normal celebrity interviews. At sports interviews you do not get massage therapists trying to convince you to sit down for a moment and enjoy a quick fifteen-minute Indian head massage. There are no shot glasses of wheatgrass juice; even at Arsenal's feng-shui-designed training ground there is just an automatic coffee dispenser and some individually wrapped chocolate bourbon biscuits. So you can imagine my response when a PR lady insisted I might like to have my boobs measured for a correct bra size. Blushing deep crimson (the mere mention of 'breast' in my more familiar work environment tends to denote a sway in conversation towards the deeply smutty), I insisted it would have to wait at least until after I had actually sat down with Mel C.

Flustered by all the offers, I wasn't sure what I'd make of Melanie (as she is now known). But, despite my cynicism, she quickly won me over. She's smiley, lovely, funny, self-deprecating, opinionated and swears like a trooper – and she didn't tell me off for asking about David Beckham. And she was stunningly beautiful. How could anyone ever have described her as the Scunthorpe United of the Spice Girls?

'I was the only one in the Spice Girls who really loved sport,' she says, instantly allaying all my suspicions. 'Victoria had to become interested in football when she met David Beckham, but for me growing up in a small industrial town on the out-skirts of Liverpool, everyone was into football. That was just how it was. Growing up, everyone I knew wore a trackie. That was Liverpool in the 1980s.' A Liverpool fan, who remembers the day of the Hillsborough disaster, the 'ashen faces' of the people behind the till at her local sweetshop that terrible Satur-day, Melanie says she loved sport at school and still loves it now. 'Sport is empowering for women,' she says. 'Look at the Spice Girls, me in a tracksuit, a global pop star, you just can't imagine it happening now, can you? I'd kill to be in a tracksuit on telly now! But we had that individuality.'

Melanie says all the Spice Girls have always kept physically fit. 'Mel B. probably trains the most out of everybody. Victoria runs, Geri does her yoga, Emma does a reluctant workout – she just hates it,' but her own obsession is triathlon. 'I was a bit scared of the idea of a triathlon at first – open-water swims, and I was scared of falling off my bike because that can really hurt. The beginning of the swim is pretty hairy because everyone's trying to get the shortest route, there's a few arms and legs and punches and kicks and things. But it's not actually that bad, the odd foot in the face is all right! I just find myself saying, "Oh sorry! Sorry! I don't want to hurt anyone." And I love my bike. It's white. Very stylish. You know the old adage, "all the gear and no idea"? Well, my triathlon trainer says, "all the kit, still shit", which very much applies to me. I'm a newbie to the sport, but I'm loving it. There's so much to it, you never get bored.'

For Melanie, taking part in sports events is not about sculpting the perfect arse, as so many women's magazines instruct us is the purpose of sport and exercise, but about the experience and the friendships that women gain from being active together. 'Being a Spice Girl we harped on about "girl power", but in the last couple of years it does feel like there's another wave of feminism going on. It's good to see, because I think "girl power" has been misunderstood at times. Empowering women is about intellect, not physical appearance. I say that because, working in the music industry, so many of our young artists – brilliant young pop artists – are so sexual. And having a young daughter I'm more aware of it than ever. I'm not criticizing anybody who chooses to express themselves in whatever way is comfortable for them, but I just think why? Why do women feel that this is how they have to express themselves? It's so sad, our society has become so obsessed with looking perfect. Everyone wants to look good, we want to look our best, but it's this constant fucking obsession, it drives me insane. I hate it. Of course, being in the public eye, in entertainment, part of my work is to look good, but when I'm in the gym – honestly, I don't care. The nice thing is that I feel there's a bit of a revolt going on, a rumble, a movement, where some women are saying they don't want to do that. They want to be known for their minds and not their bodies.'

I sit back and take a breath. Melanie has blown me away with what she has to say. We were always told that 'girl power' was meant to be a movement, but it didn't feel like it at the time; to my ears it always sounded a little infantilizing. Perhaps, as Melanie suggests, I was one of those who misunderstood what the intended meaning of that slogan really was. Or maybe I just wasn't the target age for it. Or maybe the media was so obsessed with the Spice Girls' bodies that they didn't allow them enough room to talk about anything else. And yet here we are, almost two decades later, and Melanie is a convincing spokesperson for this issue. And she's right, of course. Women have to be allowed to exist without being defined by their bodies, without constantly obsessing over them. And we have to cultivate a healthy relationship between our bodies and our minds; one that ain't all about the ass.

Maybe I underestimated the cultural impact of the Spice Girls. Maybe I took it for granted at the time. Melanie nods. 'I look back now at what the Spice Girls achieved, what we represented, and I think, "Oh, my God." We didn't fully realize it at the time, we were just five young women living our dream. But all these years later and people are still telling me that we inspired them, we made them feel it was OK to be different, it was OK to be a tomboy, it was OK to be whatever you wanted to be. I don't think we have that now for young girls.'

By the end of the interview I love Melanie. She has reinvigorated my belief in the world. If even a multimillionairess cares about girls and PE at school, about body image, about mums riding shopper bikes at triathlons, then maybe there is some hope. Maybe, even with all that money and fame, people can still care about the issues that are shaping women today, and the women of tomorrow. And that's important, because when I was a kid I don't think many people truly believed that it mattered whether a girl liked sport or not.

Melanie has put her finger on an important point: there is a revolution going on. Women are fed up of all this compartmentalizing nonsense where we are stuck into decorative, detached and sexualized roles. We want a stake in our own destinies! And whether it's Lena, or Melanie or Serena, this is a movement that is happening across the globe, in every sphere. Crucially, sport is a major part of it.

Take that Always viral *#LikeAGirl* – a short film questioning why doing anything 'like a girl' should ever, ever be seen as a lesser thing. It's so powerful it moved me to tears. Seriously, watch the tiny girl in crocs and flouncy skirt sprint across the stage in demonstration and then speak so earnestly into the camera to say, 'Run like a girl means . . . [*dramatic pause*] . . . run as fast as you can.' Too right. I want *her* to run for president. Meanwhile the current actual US president has lit up my life with a single phrase. 'Playing like a girl,' said Barack Obama as he celebrated the US women's football team World Cup win, 'means you're a badass.'

But unless we get our girls and women playing sport, or being physically active, we risk not making badass, we risk celebrating a cool phrase but never truly experiencing it beyond the rhetoric. Because the inescapable truth is that, while there are pockets of change to be found, we still have a major inactivity epidemic in the UK. Around 40 per cent of sixteen-year-old girls in this country do no vigorous physical activity. That hardly surprises me. As a sixteen-year-old I did no vigorous physical activity, unless you count blagging my way into the Camden Palace on a Tuesday night and having a dance. There was no emphasis on exercise being important to keep you healthy. No one mentioned heart rates and bone density, core strength supporting your skeleton, varicose veins, osteoporosis or arthritis. No one mentioned 'skinny fat' and what's really going on with your body inside. And there was no accountability. When I sat down in front of my PE teachers on parents' evening, they looked at me, bemused: what was I doing there? Meanwhile my recent request to see statistics from Sport England regarding physical activity and young women in the 1990s lead to a dead end: the data that monitors these things only goes back to 2005. No wonder we have such a problem.

These days, of course, we have a much greater awareness of all these health issues. But a commitment to Nutribullet and a gym session might not be the catch-all solution it is so often billed as, because too much of our health rhetoric is still fixated around body image. You've only got to flick through Instagram's fitspo hashtag to see that among the kale-eating, strength-promoting positive messages, there is also a worrying leaning towards yet another version of seeking perfection in women's bodies, an aesthetic valued higher than the internal sense of well-being it often claims to be connected with. Ultimately we still need to change our attitude to sport and the place it occupies in our lives, and this needs to start right at the very beginning – at primary school.

It was pushing my daughter on the swing the other day that crystallized things. Through the fence we watched primary-school-age boys take part in an after-school football coaching session. The more I watched, the more depressed I became. Not because there weren't any girls taking part – although that in itself is pretty sad considering that the Football Association has now lifted the gender restrictions on kids playing football together – it was more than that. I focused on the coach. A young man with a clipboard and a whistle. The only thing this football coach ever said was, 'Unlucky!' or 'Arghhhh!' Around half the class didn't receive any kind of comment, or grunt, at all.

It was heartbreaking, watching the kids who ran up to kick the ball knowing full well they had already been written off as crap. Many were half-hearted in their efforts, and their teacher barely acknowledged their existence. It was all too familiar. From such a young age we brand kids as sporty or not sporty. Fall into the wrong category and you are *persona non grata* to the average PE teacher. This could not be allowed to happen in any other curriculum subject. A teacher is obliged to help you learn, to help you to improve, to give you advice, to tell you where you are going wrong. How is 'Arghhhh!' an acceptable comment? What can any young footballer learn from 'Unlucky'? No wonder England can't win the World Cup.

A few weeks later, by coincidence, we watched the same PE teacher instruct a mixed class of boys and girls. He was sensitive around the girls, a softer voice. But there was a resignation about his demeanour. He didn't seem to believe that the girls were worth investing in. He gave them faint praise, when – quite frankly – they were terrible. They didn't seem to believe him, either, because his comments led to no discernible change in their technique. What made me saddest of all was seeing the girls' bodies over the ball, crumpled, hunched over, shying away from the task. There was no confidence in their frames.

Our school sport system doesn't seem to be working for anyone right now, girls or boys. Far too much coaching appears to be stuck in the 1980s, the same archaic attitudes that I encountered at school. I don't want to shoot down PE teachers; I imagine their lives are already hard enough as it is. Their subject isn't prioritized, isn't taken seriously enough, isn't allocated enough time in the curriculum. And from what I hear, female PE teachers in particular aren't always supported in the PE environment, with girls' PE all too often seen as secondary to boys' PE. One friend, a teacher, tells me the story of when their head of PE handed in his notice. 'As soon as he walked out the room, one of the male PE teachers turned to the head of boys' PE and said, "Well, that's good news for you, then." "Yeah," said the head of boys' PE, "and you could take over my job." All the while completely ignoring the fact that the head of girls' PE was sitting with them. When she was privately asked if she would apply for the post she said she didn't think there was any point: "I know I won't get it." When, finally, female colleagues within the department convinced her to go for the job, she was told that they wouldn't be accepting job applications for the moment as the head of boys' PE would automatically be interim head until the new school year. PE is such a boys' club, it's ridiculous. But that's the kind of shit that happens in school. Women aren't taken seriously for the senior roles. I've heard other schools talk about the same issues. The male PE teachers go out for "boys' drinks", but they don't invite the female PE teachers.'

Such attitudes are damaging and leave a legacy that can carry over into adulthood. When I quiz my friends about their PE experiences, so many of them have incredibly vivid memories, even twenty-five years on. My friend Kate recalls the male PE teacher who told her that there was no point in teaching girls to throw because they are inherently bad at it (something to do with their breasts getting in the way, he reckoned). 'It has stayed with me for life,' she says. In Kate's case I think it probably made her more determined to excel as a woman in the world, but she never did take up sport. And the wider point is that to tell young girls there are things they cannot be good at because of their biology sets up a terrible precedent for the rest of their lives. What else, those girls must wonder, am I not able to do because of my breasts?

The problem is that these sorts of attitudes about female ability, and equality, are still around in male-dominated PE departments. My teacher friend remembers a row over equal prize money in tennis, which shocked her to the core. 'I remember watching Wimbledon the first year that the women were given equal prize money [in 2007]. I said to the men in the PE department, "Isn't it brilliant? About bloody time! Can you believe it's taken this long?" and they went really quiet. So I said, "But why has it taken this long?" And they told me it is because men work harder than women, because men play five sets and women only play three. I said, "Are you serious? Are you taking the piss? Come on, boys, let's get a round, you lot are fucking jokers, ha ha." Anyway, turns out they weren't joking. They actually don't believe that women should get equal prize money. I said, "Do you think women train less than men? Do they put in less time than the men? No? So why should they get less prize money?" And some of these men are really lovely, totally unstereotypical PE teachers, sensitive, thoughtful guys. I was like, shame on you! So I took the debate and shared it with all the other PE teachers across the whole borough when we gathered together to watch the final. I said to them, "Fucking hell, can you believe this about the PE staff at my school?" Anyway, turns out they all felt exactly the same way. All the male PE teachers, to a man, from across the borough, all thought women shouldn't get equal prize money. I was on my own with it. Sorry, but what year are we in?' Of course, female tennis players themselves are open to the idea of playing five sets to earn equal prize money – as the former Women's Tennis Association CEO, Stacey Allaster, said in 2013, 'All you have to do is ask us.'

But the mood across my friend's PE department isn't an isolated one; PE seems dreadfully archaic at a time when the rest of society is moving pretty fast. The call for PE to reform is getting louder and louder, from greater flexibility over the kinds of sport covered, to demanding more time to be allocated to PE lessons full stop. Because while we're asking adults to do 150 minutes of exercise a week, we're not asking kids to do the same. Surely if we want to prepare them for a healthy lifestyle then we need to engender the habit before they grow up? The reality right now is that kids do two hours of PE a week. But once you've subtracted the time needed to get changed, listen to and follow instructions from the teacher, pack up again and get changed back into normal school clothes, you're looking at a maximum of two sessions of half an hour each.

Baroness Tanni Grey-Thompson, Britain's most decorated Paralympian turned peer, is concerned. 'PE needs a revolution,' she says in her typically refreshing, forthright way. 'PE needs to be given the same status as literacy and numeracy. We don't teach physical literacy. We teach phonics to teach people to read: the same should happen with physical literacy – jump, throw, catch, hop, skip.' I love this idea – particularly for young children. A friend of mine sends her four-year-old daughter to a scheme called Playball Kids, aimed at two- to eight-year-olds. She discovered it after an attempt to get her daughter into football failed spectacularly – the football sessions were almost all boys, and her daughter said they were too noisy and aggressive. Playball Kids doesn't focus on any one particular sport or gender, it's just about children getting the general skills they need to be physically active, with the emphasis on enjoyment. As Tanni says: jump, throw, catch, hop, skip. But only parents who can afford schemes like that, or live in areas where they operate, will have access to them. For the rest of us it's a lottery.

Tanni hits the nail on the head, and echoes my own school experiences twenty-five years ago, when she says, 'You might not like maths but you know you have to do it. You might not like PE but you can get out of it. If it were up to me I'd be more dictatorial about PE. I think we should be doing it every day in school – but delivered properly.' At St Ninian's primary school in Stirling there's a brilliant version of Tanni's utopia in action. Every day the whole school walks, runs, skips or jogs a mile-long circuit around the perimeter of the school, in addition to regular timetabled PE. It's a cost-free response to a problem that sees two-thirds of primary school children lacking basic fitness, when obesity experts recommend children exercise for an hour a day to stay healthy.

If able-bodied children are failing this target so miserably, how much worse does it get for disabled children? Tanni sighs. 'Well, they're still being excluded from PE at school and sent to the library,' she says. 'And if you're the parent of a disabled child you're probably fighting for education, benefits, healthcare, a wheelchair, childcare – so physical education is probably bottom of the list; by the time you're fighting for PE you've probably given up. There's a lot we could do to be more inclusive.'

The thing is, if we can't get PE right for young children, a captive audience obliged to take part, then how on earth can we ever expect to nail it for adults? If even at its very first hurdle sport is failing our children, how can we hope to truly effect cultural change? Sometimes it feels as though we're searching for solutions when they already exist; we just don't think to look in those places. Take the example of the Muslim Women's Sport Foundation (MWSF). Most people would assume that their expertise is only relevant to Muslim women and girls, marginalized by mainstream society. But speaking to their chair, Rimla Akhtar, proves a revelation as she tells me about schemes run for her community that would translate brilliantly into any mainstream setting. It is a stark reminder of how we casually pigeonhole people.

Minority communities undoubtedly have their own specific challenges to getting women and girls active; Rimla tells me, for example, that few faith schools have dedicated sports halls. Meanwhile the sports sector fails to reach out to communities and demonstrate that sport is a safe space for their daughters. But when Rimla describes the MWSF's six-week coaching programme that sends dedicated sports coaches into schools to work specifically with groups of teenage girls, it sounds like exactly the sort of thing that would work in any school. 'That six-week coaching programme is enough to change a girl's attitude to sport. It's about knowing that someone's coming in to focus on you and give you the attention you deserve. That's all, as a human being, that you'd want anyway. To know you're important in that frame of reference. You are wanted in the sports industry. It just takes the smallest intervention, for someone to say, "We do want you to be part of sport." That can make such a major difference. Those girls didn't want the six weeks to end.' Rimla's talking about sport here. Girls liking sport. I think too often we forget that girls can like sport; we are not biologically programmed to detest it, we are – in the main – conditioned against it. But shouldn't we try to change that?

It's a subject that, as mother to a young daughter, I feel passionately about. And I'm not the only one. Even friends who aren't greatly interested in sport have asked me what they can do for their young daughters to prevent history repeating itself when it comes to school sport. My friend, sports broadcaster Jacqui Oatley, is not leaving anything to chance. She is determined to ensure that her daughter has a better experience of sport than our generation encountered. 'I think about it every day,' laughs Jacqui. 'Poor little thing, she's only four! But I plant little messages in her mind. I want sport to be normal for her, so I take her to early years classes where she can be physically active and she loves it. I think it's really important that from a very early age sport is normal for girls to do.'

For Jacqui, helping her daughter to be confident about sport and her body is about more than just being decent at PE. It's about giving her the fundamental tools to be an empowered person, to make her own decisions, to find her own path. 'I try to sow the seeds in her mind that she can do anything if she works hard for it, little tiny messages, bite-size ones that she can understand at her age, about needing to do things for herself and not waiting to be asked. And that even if her friends don't want to do it, it doesn't matter, if she wants to do it she can. The earlier you get those messages in their minds, hopefully the easier it will be for them growing up. Not just about sport, or football, but about everything.' Jacqui is so right about this. I watch the little girls in my daughter's nursery and, mostly, they are so confident. They express their opinions, they know what they want to play with, what they feel. Why does this confidence evaporate as they grow?

I think I know. While the experts fanny about discussing whether we might entice teenage girls into PE if we supply them with enough hairdryers, or 'feminized' activities such as Zumba or cheerleading, I personally feel that one of the most central issues to this whole debate is being ignored. Because girls are not the problem. Twelve-year-olds are not inherently diva-esque madams who require the equivalent of a PE rider and an exercise entourage. The real problem here is a massive elephant in the room: our own culture. Our social values, our media – so influential on impressionable young girls – that have been allowed, for millennia, to send out this powerful, alienating message about girls and sport: that sport is unfeminine, that sport makes you sweaty and muscular, that sport is swearing and violence, that sport is ugliness in a world where women's sole priority, value and focus should be beauty and becoming an object of desire. At the time of puberty, when society is telling girls to prioritize morphing into a sex siren ASAP, is it any wonder that girls aren't buying into school sport?

So how do we fight this thing? For a start we need good PE teachers who are empowered to teach girls how to enjoy sport and exercise. Who aren't treated as second-class citizens to boys' PE teachers, and who are given enough time in the curriculum to get to know their students and work out what they like and don't like. PE teachers who can *teach*. Who can encourage a girl – or boy – to enjoy and improve in a sport, irrespective of their natural athleticism. And if we can find these happy, motivated, communicative, encouraging PE teachers then we can get rid of those arsey, sarcastic ones I remember from my youth. The power-crazed, sadistic interrogators who loved to terrorize pubescent girls about their periods, gleefully doling out unwieldy-looking store-cupboard tampons. Because no one needs those kind of PE teachers. Not girls, and not boys. Not when I was growing up. And certainly not now. Because Zumba and yoga and cheerleading are all great, and I'm totally up for offering them to girls (and boys) in a bid to get them active, but not if the message is: we're doing this because we don't think you're really going to like sport. Not if it's some sort of apologetic last-ditch attempt to get girls active at any cost. Surely it's our job to make sport attractive? To make being competitive a comfortable and fun experience, not a persecutory Darwinian exercise in weeding out the weak from the strong? Competition is a lifelong skill that we all need, and that I believe we all possess, just maybe not in the way it's been packaged to us so far, as some kind of terrifying product of the uber-macho. Society has constructed sport to appear this way; our job is to reinvent that message, not reinforce it.

To do so we need investment. In the same way that US sport has benefited from the 1972 introduction of Title IX, forcing all educational institutions to invest equally in boys' and girls' education across all subjects – including sports – the UK and other countries would do well to adopt a similar approach. And we need to *show* girls what a sporty woman looks like. We need to bust all the myths about how playing sport is unfeminine, and uncool, about the exact body shape you need to be sporty. We need to provide girls with role models – even if the media won't. Drag all those inspirational female sports stars back to their schools and colleges to speak to the next generation. Show girls their own versions of Wayne Rooney, Lionel Messi, LeBron James, Alastair Cook, Lewis Hamilton and Amir Khan. And allow them to try out any sport they like, not just the supposedly 'feminine' ones.

Sport and exercise in its most basic form shouldn't be rocket science. It should just be fun, the fundamental movement of a person's body from A to B, with a giggle and a breathless cackle at C. Because when a kid rolls down a hill they don't complain, 'Oh my Gawd, this is SUCH hard work, and my arse is still *huuuuuge*,' they enjoy it. Their brains haven't yet been indoctrinated to think that moving their bodies is a chore, or something they're 'just not that into'. How can anyone not be into moving their bodies? It's an essential requirement of life, which has absolutely nothing to do with being male or female.

That's why we urgently need to stop the rot. We need to show our kids, and ourselves, that moving your body – beyond gyrating and cleaning – is for women and girls as much as it is for men and boys. We need to teach them that their bodies are their own, not merely vessels for saucy Snapchat pics, but useful, strong, powerful aids to being a successful woman in the modern world. We need to prove to them that being physically active is not scary, it's just a natural part of life, as normal as picking your nose, or brushing your hair. We need to do this *now*. And empower the next generation to finally reclaim sport, and their bodies, for themselves.

2

Sweating is so hot right now!
Why our twenty-first-century
obsession with exercise is all wrong

I'll never forget the first time I saw a naked woman that wasn't my mum. I was twelve, she was a grown-up and standing in the showers at Park Road swimming pool, North London, soaping her pubic hair into a lather. I don't remember anything about her face, just her body: sinewy with some wobbly bits, and a big bush down below. Swimming pool changing rooms have always been instructive; one of the few places where you see naked women. Real ones, I mean, just going about their business, getting changed, or having a wash.

At the time the sight of women unapologetically displaying their bodies prompted giggles, embarrassment and the odd sneer of derision from me and my school-age friends. As a twelve-year-old I generally interpreted those women as 1970s exhibitionist feminist types making some kind of explosive political gender statement with the aid of shower gel and uninhibited pubes. Sadly, I'm not sure how many women (or men) ever grow out of that opinion. Certainly for pubescent girls, showing any part of your naked body is anathema – which made getting undressed in a public changing room challenging. It was an unspoken rule that you had to undress without anyone catching sight of your body. Welcome to the impossible world of teenage logic!

Even today, getting dressed with minimal reveal is a process deeply etched on my unconscious. Here's the drill: *1)* Fasten bra under T-shirt by pulling both arms in. *2)* Under cover of said T-shirt, drag bra around to the front of your body and hoist over boobs with minimum jiggling. *3)* Reach out under T-shirt stretching out arms into new T-shirt you want to transfer into. *4)* Discreetly whip first T-shirt off while simultaneously whipping new T-shirt on. This manoeuvre involves two challenging over-the-head moves in short succession and, if done wrong, can leave you trapped between two T-shirt neck-holes, arms flapping, belly and bra exposed to the world. *5)* Finish off with a flourish of deodorant under each armpit. *6)* Sit down and have a breather; you've earned it.

The lengths we go to not to expose our bodies is extraordinary. The irony, of course, is that women's bodies are constantly on display in the public sphere. And yet we remain so uncomfortable about revealing our bodies, even in a private setting. This, no doubt, perpetuates the recurring women's magazine topic: how to work up the courage to undress in front of your partner with the lights on. That there are women who have been married for years still unable to show their bodies to their partners makes me desperately sad. The crazy thing is that in shunning this safe female space – specifically a female changing room – an important reality check is absent from our everyday lives. Namely, that boobs and bums really do tend to look like the wobbly things I first saw at the Park Road pool all those years ago, not the pneumatic weaponry depicted daily in the mainstream media. They also tend to be accompanied by a fascinating panoply of pubic hair which, if you are to believe the images we see every day, is an endangered species in the twenty-first century.

Female body image, and its associated woes, is currently one of the biggest obstacles holding women back in the western world. It is also one of the biggest contributing factors preventing women from being physically active in the first place. A recent Sport England report found that 75 per cent of the women they surveyed wanted to take part in sport but were inhibited by fear of being judged on their appearance and ability. The study also highlighted that one in five men think sporty women are 'not feminine'. Cruelly, our own messed-up ideas about body image are preventing us from doing the one thing that could liberate us all.

Whenever I've asked men about this subject, though many confess to their own body insecurities, they seem much more relaxed. They talk about changing rooms after football practice, where teammates comfortably stroll around naked and occasionally spank each other with a towel for a laugh. They seem to know what each other's bits look like, and are happy to stand next to each other peeing into urinals.

But perhaps that's because men's bodies aren't routinely sexualized in pretty much every context, from cars to cereal packets, news stories to celebrity appearances. And that point of difference matters, because we have reached a place where we are now so bombarded with this stuff that it seems normal. Take advertising: we consume between 400 and 600 ads in their various forms each day; women's bodies feature so frequently it's almost funny. Try googling 'sexist ads' and you will find everything from cleavage selling sliced mushrooms in brine, to a US commercial in which food writer Padma Lakshmi locates an erogenous zone in a $6 burger. And it's making us unhappy. In a *Glamour* magazine report, 97 per cent of women said they had one or more negative thoughts about their body every single day and that on average, women had a negative thought about their body every waking hour of the day.

Sport is such an obvious natural combatant to all this sexy-fungi-and-burger-sauce-orgasming weirdness. Because when a person plays sport to the best of their ability they cannot possibly think about pouting for the camera. Or any other sexualized oddity. With sport you are simply, wonderfully, in the moment. Think about it: how often are women depicted actually doing something? How often do we see women being powerful, in a non-sexualized way, demonstrating purpose, strength and grit? In an experiment in 2014, No More Page 3 (a campaign group challenging the *Sun* newspaper's forty-year-old practice of publishing daily photos of topless models on page 3) trawled six months of photographs in the *Sun* and found zero pictures of women actually playing sport. Meanwhile, beyond the sports pages, women were portrayed as some kind of sexualized still life, while men were typically shown being active. And this message about gender stereotypes and expectations is so hard-wired into our brains that when we do come across images of women playing sport, they look quite – well – weird. Their faces are all messed up. Their brow is wrinkled. Their mouth is grimacing. Their hair is sweaty. Their arms are muscular. And what is incredible about the experience of viewing these images – what is so powerful, and makes me want to plaster them across every billboard in London – is that they tell a story about women that we have never really seen before. They tell a story that encapsulates everything I want my daughter to aspire to, all of the qualities I want her to have. They show women being inspirational, determined, focused, strong, unstoppable. They show women achieving, winning, celebrating, enjoying themselves, unburdened by social norms, unselfconscious.

But if women who play sport are occupying this liberated space then we have to back them up. We have to make sure that when they step off the field of play they are not made to feel like unconventional weirdos. Unfortunately, as a society we are so used to the image-obsessed narrative that even sportswomen buy into it. Take thirteen-year-old baseball sensation Mo'ne Davis, the first-ever girl to pitch a shutout in the Little League World Series. In the summer of 2014 Mo'ne became an overnight star – Michelle Obama was tweeting about her, she knocked Kobe Bryant off the front cover of *Sports Illustrated* (the first time a Little League player of either gender has made the front cover), and Spike Lee made a moving documentary about her. An ordinary African American girl from a low-income household in Philadelphia, with a phenomenal athletic talent, effortlessly beating the boys and redefining the old stereotype of throwing like a girl. Watching the film, you can't help but cheer when Mo'ne says, 'I throw 70mph, that's throwing like a girl.' Bam! Meanwhile a Philadelphia city councillor tells the anecdote of two young boys arguing over who can pretend to be Mo'ne when they throw balls at each other. Boys aspiring to be like a girl? That's powerful.

And yet, an exchange with Spike Lee when the film-maker

asks her how she feels about the *Sports Illustrated* cover leaves a telling reminder of how we are teaching our young girls to see themselves. Holding up the historic cover – an action shot of Mo'ne, ball in hand – she says, 'Just to, like, see my face on here is pretty cool, but not the face that I'm making—'

Spike interrupts. 'You don't like your face on the cover?' he asks, incredulous.

'I mean I look like a blowfish,' says Mo'ne, 'but otherwise it's pretty cool. You can see how much power I put into it.'

And that's the thing. Mo'ne's first comment is about how her face doesn't look good because she is puffing out her cheeks with the effort of her throw; her second comment is about how powerful her sporting talent is. Why are we teaching young girls to care first about how they look, and second about their talent? This girl made history, and she cares about how her face looks? That's so wrong. I think we should feel outraged about that. I think we need to change the world so that girls like Mo'ne bask in their achievements, and don't feel the need to critique their beauty. Because when Kobe Bryant is making the front cover of *Sports Illustrated* no one's going, 'Eww, you can see Kobe's armpit hair while he's hitting that slam dunk,' or 'Kobe might have just won the Championship, but he's pulling kind of a weird expression right there.' That's because, as a man, Kobe's talent is discussed first. The fact that he's also a handsome man, making him even more marketable, is just a bonus.

With sportswomen, damningly, it's too often the other way around. Some of the biggest female earners in the sports world are paid more for their marketability than for their talent. Perennial tennis underachiever Anna Kournikova is the most famous example. But the Kournikova effect is not entirely unique. In 2014 the greatest active female tennis player Serena Williams (then with eighteen Grand Slam titles) earned half the amount in endorsements of Maria Sharapova (five Grand Slam titles) – $12m. to Sharapova's $23m. In fact Sharapova's endorsements alone are so high that they dwarf Williams's total income of $20m. for the year. Money talks. And what this money is telling us is that women become rich and powerful when they conform to society's narrow ideals of beauty. Talent comes second.

In the summer of 2015, in an interview with the *New York Times Magazine*, Serena finally responded. 'If they want to market someone who is white and blond, that's their choice. I have a lot of partners who are very happy to work with me, I can't sit here and say I should be higher on the list because I have won more. I'm happy for her [Sharapova], because she worked hard too. There is enough at the table for everyone. We have to be thankful, and we also have to be positive about it so the next black person can be No. 1 on that list. Maybe it was not meant to be me. Maybe it's meant to be the next person to be amazing, and I'm just opening the door. Zina Garrison, Althea Gibson, Arthur Ashe and Venus [Williams] opened so many doors for me. I'm just opening the next door for the next person.'[4] As someone who has been routinely portrayed as difficult, arrogant, rude and aggressive, her words are truly eye-opening. The generosity of what she says is enormous, almost beyond comprehension.

But 'Maybe it was not meant to be me'? Those words haunt me. So it was with joy that I came across a comment piece from the excellent US sports journalist Dave Zirin entitled 'Serena Williams is Today's Muhammad Ali'.[5] Rather than defend

Serena against the racist and sexist bullets routinely sent her way, he set out to celebrate her for being the incredible athlete she truly is:

'. . . For years people have asked who would be, "the next Muhammad Ali." If we dare to lift our heads, it will be clear that she is right in front of us . . .'

At first, the assertion feels like sacrilege. Ali is Ali. But while Zirin concedes that many will find the comparison controversial, he pointedly dismantles every argument against why this should be so. And he's right. Not only has Serena obliterated every major rival in her field over the last decade, she's been politically active and vocal on issues as far-reaching as poverty, racism, sexism, equal pay, menstruation and police oppression. And she's done it without the support of a nation.

'. . . Not even Ali had to achieve in an atmosphere as inhospitable as Serena's athletic setting. This is about the very particular intersectional oppression she has faced as a black woman. This iconic body she proudly inhabits – her shape, her curves, her musculature – has been the subject of scorn, regardless of the results. Even at his most denigrated, Ali's loudest detractors conceded that his physical body was a work of athletic sculpture. As a man – a black man – he was objectified with a mix of admiration, longing, and envy, in the ways black male athletes have always been seen since the days of plantation sports. It was his mind and mouth that truly made him threatening. People wanted Ali to "shut up and box" for years before finally stripping him of his title.

But as that phrase implies, they still wanted him to box. Not Serena. Instead, she has had to face a tennis world that has made it clear in tones polite and vulgar that it would be so nice if she wasn't there . . .'

The way society has responded to the presence of Serena Williams is extraordinary, and outrageous. Commonly mocked as masculine and overly muscular, to the point where David Frum, editor of the *Atlantic* and a former advisor to George W. Bush, recently accused her on the basis of her appearance of using steroids, she's been called a 'gorilla' and a variety of other racial slurs more times than anyone can count. Watching her play, seeing her pose for photos and appear in commercials, I just don't get it. When I see Serena I see a goddess of a woman. In the Beats by Dre advert where she flexes the muscles in her arm, in her back, showing off the strength of her core, rippling, strong, sweaty curves – she's beautiful. I don't understand what other people are seeing when they say she looks like a man. I can only think that those opinions are born out of prejudice. For in Serena's case, more than any other prominent female tennis player, she faces an additional, aggravated dimension: race. Serena's body, her blackness, is treated as a freak show. But whereas the term 'freak' is used with reverence for the likes of Usain Bolt, when applied to a sports*woman*, it takes on an altogether more disturbing meaning.

Ask a sportswoman. In a recent poll of Britain's elite female athletes by BT Sport, 67 per cent said they feared that the public and the media valued their appearance over their sporting achievements. They thought how they looked was more important to the public than the medals they won? Society has a lot of apologizing to do. Meanwhile, over 89 per cent said they could relate to British Olympic swimmer Rebecca Adlington's *I'm A Celebrity* reality TV meltdown over her body image insecurities, and 76 per cent said the same concerns had influenced their diet and training regimes. Now these are the women who do an eye-watering number of abdominal crunches every day. Who do hill runs in the icy, wet winds of December. Who bench-press. If *they* feel pressured, what hope is there for the rest of us?

Among these amazing athletes, double Olympic gold-medallist Rebecca Adlington stands out for her particular body image anxieties. Just months after she shot to fame at the Beijing Olympic Games in 2008 I interviewed her for a cover feature in *Observer Sport Monthly*, which involved photographing her in a vintage swimsuit. She looked beautiful, but she was nervous about showing her body in front of the camera. 'It feels a bit "Oh my God,"' she said at the time. 'You feel like they [the photographer] must have shot so many gorgeous skinny people and then they've got to work with someone that's not; it must be difficult for them to get the right angle, they try and shoot their ideas and then they realize you're not skinny and it doesn't quite work.'[6]

Many have characterized Adlington as horribly insecure, but her experiences are instructive. While there has been a huge upward trend in women's magazines and lifestyle sections telling women it is OK to exercise, the vast amount of it remains rooted in beauty mythology. By that I mean the reverent tones (and tomes) devoted to female celebs who beast their bodies in the gym these days. Don't get me wrong, there is some gratifying progress going on here; the days when Madonna headed out for a run in Hyde Park without make-up and made the ten o'clock news are over. In the twenty-first century women are openly celebrated when they work on their bodies: sweat patches triumphantly circled on paparazzi photos of our most 'stunning' female celebrities. And the harder they work, the more we admire them. Whether it's the pre-holiday bikini workout, or the post-baby Bikram yoga sessions. Because exercise = perfection. Doesn't it?

Putting aside the fact that this equation is just another version of the worn-out idea that women's bodies have to strive for acceptance, the message that exercise and sport creates a particular body shape is propaganda – i.e. it's actually just not true! Small waist, toned arms, pert bottom, wobble-free thighs and perky breasts: it is a myth that if only we did more exercise we would look this way. If we worked harder and did more tricep curls, we would lose our bingo wings. If only we followed Victoria Beckham's reported regime of doing 500 sit-ups a night alongside husband David, we too would have the perfect waist. For some women that might happen. For most of us, however, it is utter bollocks. Think about it: my arms are big, ergo my arm-to-body ratio is always going to be big vs (relatively) small. I can diet until I keel over, and my arms will still be bigger than I want them to be. There's literally nothing I can do short of liposuction and stapling to achieve the kind of body that we are told to aspire to.

So thank you, Rebecca, with your honesty, your girl-next-door down-to-earth personality. Because while when Rebecca talks about her body it makes for upsetting reading, spelling out all those *Glamour* readers' daily insecurities in one fluid breath, it is also a true reflection of the limitations of our bodies. That even when we train them to an Olympic gold-medal-winning standard, they still might not look like the lady in the Special K advert. All bodies are different, all bodies have their own individual way of reacting to the work we make them do. As Rebecca so refreshingly explains: 'I've got man shoulders. Honestly . . . I look odd, I look like a Kellogg's' character, one of those mini things where their heads and shoulders are so big and then go into a "V". I can't fit into a dress or clothes, I've got this armpit hanging which is my pec muscle [she says grabbing her pectoral] that just hangs over because it's so big. I've got massive bingo wings. When we go away as a team and we go sunbathing I'm one of the bigger girls on the team. I don't have a flat stomach or anything. Mine's quite podgy, I've got the bits, the hang, the tyre,' she says, grabbing a roll of flesh from her stomach. 'And all the other girls are, like, so skinny. Literally nothing rolls over. It is quite difficult.'

Rebecca's honesty is liberating, but also sad – particularly because much of her angst has been provoked by a constant stream of media criticism and commentary relating to her appearance. The controversial Scottish comedian, Frankie Boyle, went on about how weird her face looked, and how she must be 'dirty in bed' because she's got an attractive boyfriend (now husband). Rebecca's treatment mirrors that traditionally meted out to any sportswoman not conforming to mainstream ideas about femininity: from the 'Amazonian' comments that have dogged Venus and Serena Williams's careers and 'mannish' former world number one Lindsay Davenport, to 'you're never going to be a looker' former Wimbledon champion Marion Bartoli. So it was perhaps not a surprise when Beth Tweddle, Britain's best-ever gymnast – a woman so talented that a move on the asymmetrical bars was named after her – was horrifically trolled during a live Twitter Q&A on Sky Sports recently. 'Pig ugly', 'slut', 'bitch', were just a few of the comments aimed at her. Sadly, it seems, women and sport are still only considered acceptable in the abstract. Like the *Sports Illustrated Swimsuit Issue*, packed with underwear models who don't play sport. Or the boxer Tyson Fury commenting that heptathlete hero Jessica Ennis-Hill 'slaps up well' when she steps off the track. If we insist on attractiveness to the male gaze being the standard mould for sportswomen, we will continue to alienate girls in their droves. And we lose the very essence of sport that is so liberating and empowering to women. Because the more women play sport, and normalize the image of a sporting female, the quicker we will get away from these reductive comments.

The subject of body image and sport reached tipping point in the UK with the bomb-drop that Jessica Ennis-Hill, the face of the London 2012 Olympic Games, was allegedly called 'fat' by a senior figure at UK Athletics. Pictures of Jess's mind-bogglingly flawless abdominals graced the front and back pages of almost every newspaper, alongside the headlines. While the general public struggled to get their heads around how such a perfectly toned athlete could be branded over-weight, other sportswomen claimed that they too had been put under pressure to lose pounds. Promising British triathlete Hollie Avil retired from the sport just months out from the Olympic Games in 2012, citing an eating disorder, a problem which she said was 'rife' in her sport, while heptathlete Louise Hazel said she had suffered similar criticism to Jess from the sport's governing body.

As a journalist, I tried to persuade others to speak out about the issue. Several British sportswomen I talked to admitted privately that they had experienced problems, but were reluctant to go public for fear of reprisals. Those defending their sport maintained that weight was not a cosmetic issue but a practical consideration for all sportswomen in order to excel at their events. The sportswomen I spoke to countered that women were more likely to experience criticism than their male teammates. Most damningly of all, they felt that many male coaches had little or no understanding of the diversity of female body types. They were being told that to compete in their event, they had to look a certain way, meet a certain weight. One sportswoman described to me how she had repeatedly broken down both mentally – suffering with depression – and physically – through under-performing and injury – as a result of attempting to meet an unrealistic weight target set by a senior coach.

In sport, where extraordinary athletes come in extraordinary shapes and sizes, the mind boggles that a coach could be so conservative about the human body. Athletics, for example, has shown us that unlikely candidates can achieve the most amazing things. Until triple world-record-holder Usain Bolt came along, sports scientists didn't believe that tall people could sprint competitively over 100m. The diminutive Jessica Ennis-Hill, at five foot four inches, defies logic in her ability to high-jump the British record – a foot above her own head. So why would we resolutely stick to old-fashioned ideas about what a female athlete looks like?

Much more importantly, it sets us up for a dangerous cultural precedent. We are teaching our children that fat is incompatible with fitness. Fat is shameful. Fat is controversial. Fat is the antithesis of what we are aiming to be. Yes, obesity, severe health-threatening weight gain, is problematic. But obesity is very different from fat. The novelist and game designer Naomi Alderman provides a cheering antidote to all this nonsense. Naomi wrote a blog on the issue after designing a fitness app. On its release she steeled herself for abuse on social media. 'I mean, a fat person talking about fitness is like a nun giving sex advice, right?' she wrote. She describes her own journey into discovering exercise, which felt pretty similar to my own and that of millions of other women around the world, except that she's very clear on one point: exercise has never lost her any weight. 'What happened was better: I started to enjoy being in my body. I felt better. I felt good. It is a very different feeling to be in a fat body that is moving a lot to one that hardly moves at all. It feels like love. As simple and as joyful as that.'

What follows is a touching love letter to her body, in its original shape and form, free from judgement. 'What I've learned is: the story I got told about what it meant to have a fat body, that it must mean that I sat around all day eating deep-fried stuffed-crust pizza and watching TV – that story just wasn't true. The story about how people who look like me hate to exercise just isn't true. It's so easy to let the media you see or the discourse you hear define who you are before you've even learned about yourself. And I bought into it for too long.

'I really love my body. It's taken me ages, but I'm there now. I love it in the way you love an old friend, someone who's always there to support you, who tries their hardest to help you do all the things you want to do and asks so little in return. My body is like a waggy-tailed dog in its excitement to accompany me on adventures. It's so thrilled to go for a walk or work out at the gym or take a nice bath or have some good sex or dance to some music or lift some heavy things or curl up in bed at the end of a long day. That's my fat body, which I have learned to love through exercise.'[7]

If fat challenges our perception of female, it was South Africa's 800m runner Caster Semenya who most stretched our understanding of gender, and ultimately what it means to be a woman in sport. After she won the world title in 2009, scandal broke as Caster was labelled 'intersex'. Fellow athletes cruelly branded her 'a man' after she won the gold medal in Berlin in a stunning time, while global media were sent into a frenzy over Caster's low vocal register and broad shoulders. The then teenager was subjected to a series of intrusive medical examinations over a period of eleven months in an attempt to define her sex organs.

The following year I was sent to cover her return to competitive racing at a low-key track meet in a remote part of Finland. On a steaming hot day in July, with bugs spawned by the surrounding lakes flitting through the air, the world's media descended on this tiny town. The resulting scene was disturbing. A small unmanned tent was the only area provided for athletes to change, and several journalists attempted to peep through the gaps in the canvas to catch a glimpse of Caster as she changed into her running gear. There were no restrictions. Everyone felt entitled – and equipped – to assess Caster's gender for themselves. Was she, or wasn't she, a man?

Caster's story taught us that gender is merely a spectrum of hormones, not a definitive model. Scientists continue to argue over the issue, but many maintain that there is no clear line between male and female, rather an expansive grey area in which a range of body types exist. A study using medical data from US births between 1955 and 1998 estimated that around one in a hundred people had body variations that differ from the standard male or female types. This includes people who appear from the outside to have so-called normal genitalia, but who may have 'abnormal' sex chromosomes internally.

Of course, sport, in its commitment to upholding a level playing field in its most traditional sense, prefers to segregate – and regulate – gender. Whispers suggested that Caster's case was not an isolated instance. Other athletes, past and present, had also been prodded and poked. Most recently, having been banned from competing at the Commonwealth Games in 2014, India's Dutee Chand was subjected to a naked examination and issued with an ultimatum: either undergo surgery or take hormone-suppressing drugs. 'I cried for three straight days after reading what people were saying about me [on the Internet],' the sprinter told the *New York Times*. 'They were saying, "Dutee: Boy or girl?" and I thought, how can you say those things? I have always been a girl . . . I was made to understand that something wasn't right in my body, and that it might keep me from playing sports,' she said.[8] Dutee stood her ground. For others, it was already too late. A study published in the *Journal of Clinical Endocrinology & Metabolism* (*JCEM*) in 2011 revealed that four female athletes at London 2012 had been taken to France and operated on to remove their testes and allow them to continue competing. Despite there being no sporting necessity to the procedures they were also given a clitoris reduction, feminizing plastic surgery and oestrogen replacement therapy.

I interviewed Caster in 2011, an experience that I found emotional. As a journalist, I was expected to ask about her gender; as a human being I felt compelled to respect her privacy.

Several weeks later I received an email from a reader. It said: 'I am the mum of a pre-teen girl with a DSD (Difference/ Disorder of Sex Development), which the popular media still often refer to as intersex. Although I am not familiar with Caster Semenya's diagnosis, the sensationalist coverage that followed her world record was observed in silent horror by the many families who have a DSD child.' The email stopped me in my tracks. I'd felt like a failure for not pursuing a line of questioning about Caster's genitalia. But after reading that email, I was glad I had held back.

Dutee bravely took her case to the Court of Arbitration for Sport. And in 2015 CAS suspended the use of 'hyperandrogenism' rules, the very edict that had prevented Dutee and Caster from competing in their natural state. CAS gave sports governing bodies two years to come up with new evidence, or face scrapping the rule altogether.

Sport is an obvious front line for these issues, and it needs to make sure it is acting responsibly for women and girls battling for the right to define their own gender, the right to define their own sense of femininity, and – fundamentally – the right just to compete. While sport can be liberating for women, too often sport has been our oppressor. From the death penalty imposed in Ancient Greece on any woman caught watching the Olympic Games, to the outright ban that existed until 1984 on women running the Olympic marathon, or the ban on women's Olympic ski jumping because of unfounded fears over the damage it could cause to a woman's reproductive organs, revoked in 2014. Even today, for women in Iran, just watching volleyball can have you thrown into prison.

Wonderfully, despite the barriers, women past and present

have fought the system. Just as we tell women today to vote, in honour of the suffragettes who campaigned for the right to do so, so we owe it to those female sports pioneers to draw inspiration from their stories, to continue their fight. One of my favourite stories is of a rebel runner by the name of Roberta Gibb. The US marathoner became the first woman to compete in the iconic Boston Marathon, in 1966, when women were not allowed. Roberta, a confident amateur runner who casually clocked forty miles in a day, hid in the bushes at the start line and then jumped out at the gun to join the men-only race. Tentative at first, she ran in disguise with a hoodie concealing her face, but, supported by the male runners around her, she slowly peeled off her layers and ran openly as a woman, defiant. Up and down the course word spread like wildfire: a woman was running in the pack! The media latched on to the story, and along the roadside spectators began to pick her face out in the crowd, and cheer.

In a moving passage from her memoir *A Run Of One's Own*, Roberta describes the reaction from the crowd as she passed Boston's famous women's arts institution, Wellesley College, midway along the route. 'They were screaming and crying. One woman standing near, with several children, yelled, "Ave Maria." She was crying. I felt as though I was setting them free. Tears pressed behind my own eyes.' Roberta was instantly struck by the weight of responsibility on her back. 'I knew that if I failed to finish I would reinforce the prejudices and set women's running back another twenty years.' Despite running conservatively she finished in a time of 3 hours 21 minutes – beating two-thirds of the all-male field. News of her achievement went global. 'It was a pivotal point in the evolution of social consciousness,' she subsequently wrote. 'It changed the way men thought about women, and it changed the way women thought about themselves. It replaced an old false belief with a new reality.'[9]

It would take another six years, though, and a stream of female impostors infiltrating the race, before women were officially allowed to compete at Boston, in 1972. And, befuddled by codswallop science about women's bodies – namely that endurance running could render women infertile – it was only in 1984 that the Olympic Games finally allowed women to compete in the marathon. One of the key figures in the effort to push the Olympic agenda was American marathoner Kathrine Switzer, who also illicitly competed in the Boston marathon, entering under her initials only so that the organizers did not know she was a woman. Ten years later, in 1977, when Kathrine was director of the US Women's Sports Foundation, Avon cosmetics approached her with an interest in sponsoring a women's marathon. It is hard to convey just what a big deal this was. Can you imagine? A cosmetics company wanting to sponsor women's endurance running at a time when female perspiration was akin to bra-burning? Despite the taboo, the partnership went ahead and the first Avon International Marathon was held the following year in Atlanta, Georgia, involving competitors from nine different countries.

An interview in the *Guardian* with Kathrine, dated 1 August 1980, portrays an extraordinary woman ahead of her time. Her slogan for the Avon series, 'The beauty of women in motion', catches on to an idea that is only just now being incorporated into the mainstream – that women doing sport is a natural fit, and something we should be celebrating joyously. Sport is not at odds with beauty. Kathrine went a step further still, and waxed lyrical about the amazing smell of sweat. 'Sweating is one of the most fantastic things that can happen to your body,' said Kathrine at the time. 'Fresh sweat doesn't smell bad at all. And I just love the smell of sweating through perfume.' Can you imagine anyone saying that now? They'd be socially excluded.

Kathrine had the whole women and body image thing cracked all those years ago. 'A woman achieves a better balanced self image [through sport and exercise],' she told the *Guardian* at the time. 'She can more easily regard men as friends and vice versa, because a common level of understanding is established. Men and women who run, play and strive for common goals together appreciate each other.' She also believed in the power of sport and exercise to promote creative and intellectual thinking, ascribing enhanced thinking qualities to the various stages of a marathon, with the final few miles enabling 'free floating fantasy. That is when people talk about a runner's high; you're almost stoned on running. You hear a car honking but it's like you're wearing a space helmet. You feel like you could run forever, with the cares of the world away from you, you become part of the Universe.'[10] With Kathrine's help we're building a picture here: exercise helps you think, it puts you on a level playing field with men, it gives you body confidence, and it even makes you smell great. What's not to love?

Under Kathrine's unique direction the marathon series grew, holding events in Germany and the UK, while behind the scenes she lobbied for Olympic inclusion, flying to Los Angeles in 1981 when the International Olympic Committee's executive board were meeting to vote on the subject. In September of that same year the IOC confirmed that a women's marathon would be included, and the inaugural race took place at the 1984 Los Angeles Games. The very first female winner was Joan Benoit of the United States, who triumphed in a time of 2 hours 24 minutes and 52 seconds – a mark that would have beaten thirteen out of the nineteen previous Olympic men's marathon finals.

Thirty years on and, though we might not think of it this way, running is still very much a feminist act. Why else did Nike name their women-only 10km after-dark race series 'We Own the Night'? A nod to the 'Reclaim the Night' feminist marches originating in 1970s Britain and America, supporting the right of women to be safe from violence and harassment at any time of day or night. The same issue of safety continues to affect female runners in the twenty-first century, who are often targeted for assault in parks and open spaces. Running, sport, exercise – in its truest form – is as much about women taking back control of their own bodies as any other feminist act.

Switch on the TV and sport might still look relatively old-fashioned, with female cheerleaders and all-male punditry panels discussing predominantly male sport, but away from the mainstream there is a revolution going on. Women are quietly finding their own entry points into sport, and what's really interesting is that they are doing it without conforming to stereotype. The idea of the 'sporty woman', as a singular type, is slowly being eroded as women are drawn to an increasingly diverse spectrum of activities. Who could have predicted that endurance events such as Tough Mudder, which involves crawling under barbed wire and through ice-cold water and mud, would be attractive en masse to women? These events were originally marketed to male audiences, but women are voting with their trainer-clad feet and bucking the trend, with the ratio of women to men changing radically.

And yet at the other end of the scale there is an increasing trend for women-only participation events. For millennia sport has been set by a male agenda; now women are beginning to define its existence for themselves. It may sound superficial, but the UK-based Cycletta series – aimed at novice cyclists – which ends with massages and beauty treatments for participants is positively revolutionary; or the Nike runs where the winner's medal is replaced by a piece of limited edition Alex Monroe jewellery for every runner who crosses the line. Women's participation is shaking up tradition, finding new avenues to explore and defying the age-old wisdom that sporting culture should never be messed with. Proof that the popularity of this approach is actually working is borne out by the numbers: in 2013 over 85,000 women across thirty-seven different countries competed in the 'We Own the Night' runs. While Active People Survey data shows that almost a million British women were running at least once a week in 2014 – equating to 3.8 per cent of the female population (as compared with 5.66 per cent of men).

Mass participation events fused with beauty treatments and fashion, like these, are the modern companions helping sport and exercise – for some women – to lose that fear factor. I'm not trying to say that sport is only palatable to women when it's dressed up in beauty and fashion, but I do think some of those markers help to create a sense of this being a welcoming space for women, whether all women find those elements necessary or not. Personally I'm not sure I really want a facial after a 50km bike ride, but if it gets another woman out of bed and onto her bike that morning then I'm praising it to the high heavens.

Of course, cynics may say that race organizers don't really care about women, and that it's just another way of exploiting female bodies. Maybe. But I'm happier seeing a company make money out of female bodies in a way that promotes a positive message to and about women, than seeing women's bodies heavily sexualized to sell everything from beer to men's sport. And I'm happy that sportswear for women is finally being recognized as something worth investing in. Several years ago I consulted for a major sportswear brand on their female customer base. At the time they sold two types of women's sports bras. And both were the sort that gave you a single boob, along with the indignity of wrestling it over your head to get it on. At that time women were definitely seen as second-class citizens when it came to sports consumerism. Fast forward nearly a decade and it's amazing to see how things have changed. I'm genuinely excited to see all the colours and styles available to women these days. It is a far cry from the era where women, including myself, routinely wore two bras just to get enough support to go for a light jog.

That women can now buy an actual proper serviceable sports bra, in an array of colours, is a step forward. Like it or not, consumerism speaks volumes about the status of gender, race and every other protected characteristic in society today. In the same way that it is now (a little bit) easier to find make-up for brown skin, indicating a degree of normalization around women of colour, it is meaningful that Puma sportswear has invested zillions of dollars in its women's sports gear by hiring pop icon Rihanna to design its clothing range. Women in sport are worth investing in.

Overall, the landscape of sport and exercise is starting to feel a lot more female. While a *Cosmo* editor was recently quoted as saying that her readers were 'scared of the word sport', women's magazines across the sector are beginning to challenge that fear and embrace the subject. *Glamour* has backed Sport England's This Girl Can campaign, celebrating women with ordinary body shapes discovering physical activity for the first time; the magazine also launched its own campaign, 'Say No To Sexism In Sport', in 2015. Meanwhile everyday features, from 'Five Top Reasons to Play Netball' (including getting to plait all your friends' hair) to the best sports bras to buy for big-breasted women, are becoming increasingly common across the top women's interest publications.

There are a myriad of reasons as to why women are exercising and competing more and more, many to do with health or fitness or losing weight. But the smart ones will have latched on to something far more valuable. That sport and exercise is fun. Not when you're worrying about losing weight, or toning your thighs, but when you're running through cold mud with your best friend and laughing your heads off at how ridiculous it all is, or exploding with joy at Zumba because you're shaking your *derrière* and you just don't care. No one tells you about the fun, though, do they? Because fun is a word that women are not taught enough about. When I watch TV with my four-year-old daughter, the adverts tell her that a new pink hairclip or shiny, sparkly shoes will be FUN! But these are lies. Hairclips are not much fun. Not compared to running around a park giggling, waving your arms, rolling down a hill, kicking up leaves, throwing sticks in a pond. That's fun for a four-year-old. Similarly, women are told that exercise and sport is all about hard work, about getting the perfect body. Grafting for those flawless abs.

Shifting that baby fat. We are not told that we might have any fun doing it. After all, this is supposed to be our penance, for having women's bodies that don't look right. Isn't it ... ? But what is this obsession with women's bodies having to be the 'right' shape, anyway? Surely the whole wonderful thing about sport is that it showcases the amazing diversity of the human body. From pint-sized US gymnast Gabby Douglas breaking race barriers to become all-around Olympic champion in 2012, to the slip-of-a-frame world and Olympic champion rower Helen Glover, or the power of New Zealand's multi world- and Olympic-medallist shot-putter Valerie Adams.

I phone my friend Kate McKenna. At the age of twenty-five she has recently taken up adult gymnastics at the same gym where Beth Tweddle trained in Liverpool. It's a scheme that has been rolled out nationally by British Gymnastics in an effort to encourage adults to return to a sport they probably won't have tried since they were kids. Each week Kate posts a video of herself on YouTube performing jaw-dropping routines. As we chat Kate confesses that it took her a whole year to work up the courage to attend adult gymnastics, which is mixed gender. 'I knew as soon as I got there that it would be fine, but I was worried about looking silly, people laughing at me. It's such a difficult age to get fit again. You're self-conscious in your twenties, I'm the least confident I've ever been – struggling to find work, having to move back in with your parents. It's not an easy time.

'In my twenties my body changed,' says Kate, describing an experience familiar to so many women of her age. 'A similar thing happened to a lot of my friends. I'd never had to worry about my weight before, but everything changed after I finished uni and I remember looking in the mirror and thinking, "This just isn't me."' Kate put herself on a carb-free diet ('the worst week of my life . . . and it didn't solve anything') and watched her body struggle to adapt to the changing demands of a twenty-something metabolism and lifestyle.

Watching Kate's YouTube videos makes my heart soar. There is this beautiful curvy young woman grinning ecstatically as she nails a full twisting somersault into the pit. Or a round-off backflip tuckback. (Yeah, I had to google it too. It's gym chat for shit-hot-wow.) I've never seen gymnastics like it. We're all conditioned to view gym as a sport for tiny teenagers. Like, if you didn't start double piking aged eleven, you can forget about it. That may be the case for someone wanting to win an Olympic medal, but just for mucking about and having a great time? Not any more. British Gymnastics are pushing the trend, and Kate loves it. 'The best thing about adult gymnastics is that it's fun,' says Kate. 'I literally spend an hour and a half messing about, playing, and the next day every single muscle in my body aches like I've done a hardcore workout.'

It took me a while to learn that exercise can be fun. I was a latecomer to the concept of being physically active. I only really started working out in my twenties, a period when my body was changing – like Kate's – and the days of eating a packet of chips on the way home from school with no obvious effect were definitely over. At the time I was at university, and I felt low. All around me everyone seemed under pressure to perform academically. Undergraduates exchanged gruesome stories about where former students had hanged themselves on the campus. There were long stretches of time on your own, with books that made your brain hurt and never seemed to make any sense no matter how many times you read them.

Finding aerobics changed everything. A chance to jump around, forget about all the weighty cerebral struggles, just physically be and nothing more. I recently heard about a leading adoption expert who insisted that the one immoveable part of his programme for adopting teenage kids was to make sure they do exercise. He says it is a make-or-break element – it's that effective in determining how they cope emotionally with adjusting to a new home. For me, the emotional tonic I needed was aerobics. What I loved most about the classes was the communal feel of it, all those grey-haired mums and grandmas busting a grapevine or a box step, shaking their hips. It was the older generation who never missed a class, who laughed most, who came with their friends, who worked the hardest. Aerobics was their lifeline: to being active, to being social, to leaving all other responsibilities aside. It was their precious time for themselves, and they loved it. Watching them, I felt inspired. But looking back I can't help wondering: why are women waiting until their autumn years to have this eureka moment? Why can't younger women find the same enjoyment?

When I left university and returned to London I had to find a new fitness regime all over again. My best friend Tamzin suggested running a 10km together and promised me I would be able to manage it. I wasn't so sure. Having been put off running for life by hellish cross-country sessions in PE, I was a reluctant runner. After a few painful jogs around the local park we set off for the British 10km Road Race on a sweltering August day in London. Halfway round I was walking. Hobbling. Swearing I would never run again. I thought that was the end of it, I was clearly a terrible endurance runner.

That's probably because I didn't yet know that running involves a degree of pain. Even at my fittest, running still makes my lungs hurt, my heart pound frantically in my chest. I wonder – in the odd paranoid moment – if I am going to die. Of course I have come to realize that is all quite normal. But encountering those sensations for the first time can be terrifying. Years later, working as a sports journalist, I listened with interest as Liz McColgan-Nuttall, Britain's distance-running luminary of the 1980s and 1990s, talked to me about relocating to Qatar, tasked with finding future female endurance medallists from a nation of girls still unfamiliar with physical exertion.[11] Qatar only started to allow women to compete at an Olympic Games in 2012. I sat spellbound as Liz described trawling Qatari girls' schools for running talent, and finding a generation of young women disconnected from their own bodies.

'They would get all worried and scared because they had never been out of breath before,' she said. 'They'd never had sore muscles or cramp, they didn't know what was happening to their bodies.' I rang my editor to give him a summary of the interview; on the other end of the phone he sounded excited. 'That's a line, isn't it?' he said enthusiastically, '"never been out of breath before", wow.' I agreed and put down the phone. In the hours that followed I realized my own idiocy. The first time I went for a run I was an adult, and I had never properly been out of breath before. Not really, you know, heaving, head pounding, lungs burning. I too had been scared by the ferocity of those sensations – was this normal? Could my body cope? Would I faint?

Was I weak? Perhaps British culture was less enlightened than I thought.

After that terrible August 10km road race I didn't think I would ever run again. But I did. Inexplicably, something, somewhere, clicked. I began to undertake tiny runs on my own in the park. No more than a mile, baby steps. Then my housemate Elaine said she'd like to join me. She had never run before, and I was thrust into the unfamiliar role of helping someone else to run. There was no aim to it. We weren't trying to lose weight, or run a race, or beat each other. We were just running for the hell of it. Together, we caught the running bug. We ran in the hot summer sunshine, we ran in the biting wind and rain, we ran in the snow (imagining ourselves as husky dogs pulling a sleigh), working as a team to get us home. We ran down London's great Regent's Canal, past corners that stank of urine, leaping over dog shit, or vomit, ignoring the drunks occupying badly broken benches. We inhaled the woodsmoke, warm and inviting, chugging out of the canal boats, and jumped out of the way of careering cyclists speeding along the banks. One cold winter's night we were chased through an estate by a group of kids armed with sticks and swear words. And every time we arrived home, gasping, burning, but exhilarated, we'd trudge up the stairs to our flat, rip off our sweaty layers and grin for the rest of the evening.

We felt great. And we talked about that feeling all the time, using it as a reminder to dare the other one to squeeze in just one more run, no matter how uninviting the circumstances (like: hungover on a breakfast of crisps and Lucozade). The one thing we never talked about was our weight, or how we looked, or what we would wear on our runs. We didn't need to. The feeling we were getting from the run overrode any other consideration that might otherwise dog us in our everyday lives. Feeling great became more powerful than looking great. And that feeling extended beyond just a post-run high on a Thursday night. That feeling had longevity, and impact. It cemented our friendship, it propelled us through career challenges, relationship break-ups, house-sharing squabbles and regrettable one-night stands. Running became a way of boosting life to a previously unattainable level. It was liberating.

Don't just take my word for it. A recent study published by the British Psychological Society focused on how exercise can change the way we view our bodies – even before any discernible physical change. Dr Katherine Appleton explored participants' feedback over a two-week period, crucially a short enough period that physical benefits would not yet begin to factor. Her conclusion that 'a focus on body image [and our responses to it] . . . may be more rewarding for those embarking on an exercise programme' is enlightening because it is a rare example of the emphasis being placed on how we feel after doing exercise, as opposed to how we look.

It was a no-brainer then that on the morning of one of the most important days of my life – my wedding – it was Elaine who came to meet me for a run, before any hairdressers or make-up artists or friends with bouquets or cameras. Off we set, as we had done so many mornings before, stretching in the September sunshine. A final gasp of unadulterated female friendship: no talking, just breathing and legs turning. 'One, two, three, four, five, six, seven, eight, nine, ten,' I counted in my head, urging my thighs to keep lifting my knees. 'Breathe in, breathe in, breathe OUT,' I puffed, nostrils noisily inhaling, mouth exhaling.

A week later, on my honeymoon, I ran with my husband through gorse bushes in the South of France. It caused the only argument of an otherwise wonderful trip. 'Come on!' he teased, 'you can run faster than that, surely?' He laughed. This was meant to be encouragement, banter. I seethed. And snapped. This male approach wasn't what I was used to. Contrary to every bitchy portrayal of women, running with my girlfriends was supportive, encouraging, caring, fun. Every time we ran Elaine would say, 'Shall we run a bit further tonight?' To which I would groan, 'Noooo! I can't! I swear I can't do it . . .' She'd nod and say, 'OK then, don't worry.' And because of her kindness, and because I didn't want to let her down, I'd buckle and change my mind. 'OK, let's do it,' I'd say, shaking my head. And then we'd run our hearts out.

Through running I found that friendship was central to exercise. It was Tamzin who convinced me to start running, against all the odds, and Elaine who helped me to keep at it even when I least felt like it. It became about teamwork, about supporting each other, about the very fundamental act of making it possible to get out – because we couldn't have run down the canal alone in the dark and still felt safe. Even better, running together meant sharing the exhilaration. And the laughter.

No matter how tired we were, at the end of the run Elaine and I always sprinted the final 100m, just for fun. It was my favourite bit. 'Ready? Steady? GO!' Somehow the energy came flooding into our legs, a whoosh of adrenaline, the excitement of sprinting, feeling like your body was being propelled by your quads, so fast you might just stumble and fall over. Sometimes we'd shout. Sometimes we'd cheer. We ran so fast it felt like flying. I have amazing female friendships, but that feeling of flying together down a ropey canal, or round the bend of a litter-strewn park, cannot be replicated. It is right up there with my best-ever moments. Thinking about it gives me goosebumps, like it did to hear my best friend talk about giving birth – a gentle soul transformed as she literally lifted the hospital bed from the pain of her contractions – or that buzz of an amazing night out dancing.

In my day job, when I interview female sports stars this is one of the recurring themes they themselves talk about: that strengthening sense of female friendship. And it's not just about having a nice bunch of friends, it's about that group dynamic and the positive lessons it gives young women. I see it especially in team sports, where women lose their inhibitions and sing and dance and loudly joke about in front of huge crowds, buoyed by their camaraderie. As a non-sports person it can be hard to understand; surely all women have great friendships? That's one of the things we pride ourselves on. But if our friendships are so great, then why aren't we helping each other to make more of them? To be physically active, healthy and happy? When I met Olympic and world champion rower Helen Glover in 2014 she talked about her close friendship with rowing partner Heather Stanning. 'When we're in the boat I want to win for her as much as for me,' she said, echoing my exact feelings about running with Elaine. After dropping out of sport, and then being identified in the talent recruitment programme, Sporting Giants, ahead of London 2012, Helen is evangelical about providing sporting opportunities to school-age kids. 'When I go to school talks now, I want to convince them they can do it too,' she says. 'The thing is you just don't think it can be you. I remember being in school assembly and they asked us, "What do you want to be when you're older?" In my head I thought, "Win Olympic gold", but I put up my hand and said, "Vet".' There's that perceptions thing again, worrying what others will think, unsupported by our environment to truly pursue our goals, afraid to voice our ambitions.[12]

But at the end of the day, how much time do we want to waste on this appearance stuff? How much more time do we really want to spend arguing over whether Kim Kardashian's naked arse is female empowerment or exploitation? All this discussion accompanying endless music videos with buttock-shaking slo-moes, selfies, belfies, conversations about implants, eating disorders, Botox and dieting, is enough to make you go mad. Or contract body dysmorphia, if you haven't already got it.

This 24/7 stream of poison that affects every female being subjected to these images, whether they are an elite athlete with the 'perfect' butt, or not. This tyrannical grip over what is feminine, and what – most importantly – is not. Because what's the alternative? The TedX make-up artist Eva DeVirgilis spells it out when she says that it takes three seconds for a woman to sit in her make-up chair and tell her what they hate about their face. That only women in their autumn years, or dying from cancer, seem to celebrate being there, enjoy the process of applying make-up as something fun, rather than something they depend upon simply to leave their house. It's a theme that women the world over are finally waking up to. Australia's Sky News anchor, Tracey Spicer, in her inspirational TedX talk that went viral, argues that we're wasting precious minutes – hours – each day on beauty routines, time that could be spent doing something more productive. Having calculated that she was spending an hour a day – or fifteen days a year – on hair and make-up, Spicer asked women to tot up how much time they spent on their beauty habits, and then work out what they could be doing instead. By the end of 2014 Spicer had dropped the fake tan, hair curlers and body-control tights.

Sport is one of our greatest opportunities to escape this constant undermining life-ruining drip feed about what women and girls should look like – in some cases even down to our genitals. Because if we embrace sport and exercise for women properly – championing female athlete role models in education and the media – then we won't have this body dysmorphia crisis. Because there won't be a 'normal' women's body, just a life-affirming brilliant array of every type of female body under the sun – boobs of all shapes and sizes, curvy hips, slim hips, broad shoulders, tiny bums, huge great powerful gluteal asses, wispy legs that travel for miles, hulking great thighs that accelerate over 100m, bellies that dance, or are neatly stacked in six-pack abdominal squares.

And once we accept that we needn't look a certain way, then we can start to share our euphoria about exercising or playing sport rather than a perfectly poised appearance, contrived post-workout pouting, critically staring into our phones. Just take the picture, and bugger the extreme red face and sweaty hair! Or maybe we don't even need to instagram every moment of our lives for others to judge. Maybe exercise and sport can be something we do for ourselves. For fun! For happiness! For clear thinking! Because physical activity should be something integral to our being alive. And it is the essential part that really concerns us here, not the bit about how many millimetres it might shave off your inside thigh measurements.

Let's be real for a moment. The outside of our bodies is only a tiny part of who we really are. When women begin to realize that physically connecting with our own bodies isn't about being bullied by a media assault of unattainable female images, then we will begin to come into our own. Maybe we will stop curling our eyelashes every day and use the extra thirty-five minutes a week to read up on nuclear physics, or maybe we will give up the frappuccinos with friends and instead meet them outside in the fresh air for t'ai chi or a kick around with a ball. Maybe we will take our sons, daughters, nieces, nephews and grandchildren to the park and RUN like the wind until we're out of breath, and laughing. And maybe then we will discover that feeling generated when women become part of a physically active community: the confidence, the friendships, the energy to take on every other challenge in our lives – from dysfunctional relationships, motherhood and the gender pay gap, to just having a really great time.

Just as women fought for the vote, and that very achievement compels us to the polling stations, so women have fought for the right to exercise and participate in sport, and we cannot throw that away. From the women of ancient Greece putting their lives on the line just by watching sport, and the women in Iran who continue to risk imprisonment today by doing the same, to the likes of Kathrine Switzer who campaigned for women to be allowed to run any distance they liked, or Caster Semenya and Dutee Chand who demand the right to participate in sport as women, without being told what their labia should look like.

We need to reclaim sport and exercise for women. It needs to become part of our world, not a borrowed space where we are allowed to intrude. We can decide ourselves what we want it to look like: whether we want all-female events, or jewellery, or beauty treatments, or crèches or free access to make sure that all economic groups can attend. Because when sport and exercise become normalized in a way that reflects society – real women doing real physical exertion free from worries about what anyone else thinks – we will be able to truly embrace our bodies. And enjoy them. After all, from pooing to prancing, periods to pregnancy, these are the real miracles our bodies perform. Not squeezing into that size 10 dress, or nailing the latest up-do. But finding our muscle, and wielding it. Just a little.

3

Why sport will make you successful

How many times have I asked for a pay rise? Once. And I nearly cried. How many times have I asked for a promotion? Never. That's the problem with so many women in the workplace, we think careers are like a 1940s tea dance. Nice girls wait to be asked. But after fifteen years of work, I'm finally realizing that men do things differently. Or so I hear. There's X who demanded to be promoted to chief whatsit, or Y who refused to take the job unless he was paid £10K more than it was advertised for. Why aren't I more like them?

According to one study that has received worldwide attention, sport has everything to do with it. In 2013 multinational firm EY found that women with sports backgrounds were more likely to reach the top of the career ladder. As journalists hurried to distribute the news, it wasn't hard for them to find real-life examples. From Hillary Clinton (college basketball), head of the International Monetary Fund Christine Lagarde (France national synchronized swimming team), Condoleezza Rice (figure skating and tennis), to Brazilian president Dilma Rousseff (volleyball) and CEO of Pepsi Indra Nooyi (cricket).

My favourite example of all time, however, has to be Twitter board member Marjorie Scardino, an ex-rodeo rider.

So what does sport give women that they wouldn't otherwise have? Of course it teaches you how to win, how to lose and how to work in a team. But according to the EY report, the most important thing sport teaches you is how to bounce back from rejection, failure and all other manner of major or minor setbacks. That's both liberating and empowering. Finally, here's a way to take on that gender pay gap in a world where women are forfeiting an average of £100,000 over the course of a lifetime.

Michelle Moore is one of those people who have benefited from sport. A former athlete who competed at county level in her youth, now in her forties she still displays all the traits of a sportswoman's drive. 'Someone said to me recently that I often refer to myself in the third person,' says Michelle. 'Apparently that's typical of ex-athletes. I'd always look for my name in *Athletics Weekly*, page 89, and keep a scrapbook of all the cuttings in which my name was mentioned.' Illeism, or referring to yourself in the third person, is a recognized trait among sportspeople – from Pelé to Andre Agassi. It's often mocked as egotistical, but research suggests that it's actually a helpful habit to have as it calms the brain and improves performance in the workplace.

'Undoubtedly sport has had a huge effect on my career,' says Michelle. 'Sport brought out my natural leadership abilities – as netball captain, as a fast runner, and as the eldest of five children, sport helped to hone who I am. In my career I've fast forwarded through every level, at every stage. I want to win. I want to be the best. I've got a really intense work ethic.' That drive translated into her career, and Michelle has been a high-flyer ever since. At thirty-two she was assistant head teacher in a secondary school, rising to become one of a very few black women in a senior position with local authority management, and is now an expert on diversity in sport. Michelle is adamant that a youth spent on the athletics track prepared her for a successful path in the workplace. 'You come to see yourself almost from the outside. I think it's a result of constantly measuring yourself against external barometers. You see yourself as a machine, an entity.'

Echoing the EY research, Michelle agrees that it's the disappointments from her sporting experiences that still motivate her today. 'I think as female leaders we have to have resilience. I'll never forget being fifteen years old, at the English Schools' Championships, my biggest-ever competition. I had to do a race-off with another girl to secure a place in the 400m final, and a chance of earning an international vest to represent England. I wanted that so badly, and yet I lost the race because I was overcome with nerves. I still feel that loss today, and I'm so annoyed with myself. It still hurts, and I still wonder what my life might have been like had I won.'

Nowadays the 'winning' is played out in her life post-athletics. During the London Olympics the local organizing committee asked council departments to get schools to sign up and secure their allocation of tickets for schoolchildren in their borough. Michelle was determined to be the first local authority in the country to get all her schools signed up. 'My motivation was about doing something great for the kids, yes, but if I'm honest what drove it all was my obsession with always wanting to be the first. I just love coming first. And it's a hidden first, because nobody actually ever knew that it was me who had achieved it. But that didn't matter, I just wanted us to be first.'

It's so rare to hear women speak openly and unashamedly about wanting to be the best at work. Despite all our societal demands for a more productive workforce and economy, being competitive is still a taboo for women – as though, somehow, it's all a bit bitchy and unseemly if you want to get ahead. Michelle nods. 'When you're ambitious people are intimidated. They want to put you down. In a management position, such as I am in, you are seen as being difficult. You know, "She's got really high standards, she needs to relax a bit." They don't get it – I get things done. That's what I'm known for.' But shouldn't ambition, or getting things done, be lauded? Maybe if more women were able to embody these qualities, and actively pursue them at work, we wouldn't have such a debilitating attitude to all this stuff.

Olympic bronze-medallist heptathlete Kelly Sotherton laughs knowingly. 'I've been called a loudmouth or an interferer, or a moaner or a troublemaker – you don't really hear people say that about a man though, do you?' says Kelly, who retired from athletics ahead of the London Olympic Games, but is living proof of the EY report's conclusions. Even as a young athlete Kelly was always upfront about her ambitions beyond her athletics career. She wanted to be a chief executive and have a say in how her sport is governed. That aim has not changed. 'I want to run my sport, one day. The ultimate goal for me is to be president of the IOC. That's a far-fetched comment but if I can get anywhere near that I'll be happy.' Now she's on the UK Sport International Leadership Programme maybe she'll make it. In the meantime she's being headhunted in the business world, and when I ask her which skillsets they see in someone who has spent her life on a training track, rather than an office, and has no experience in business, her answer is illuminating.

'When I went to see the managing director of one company, he said: you have every attribute I'd like in someone coming to work with me. Someone who can succeed and plan and perform; they're the same skills you need in business, it's just learning a bit more business acumen. But you've learned and coached and can take direction, be critiqued and learn to use that to your advantage – as a sportsperson you're not offended by criticism, you just use it to improve, and that's a skill that I think a lot of people who haven't been in sport don't have. They don't like to be criticized because they think it's offensive. But if it's constructive, it's something you can learn from and it helps you to improve your performance. I spoke to various people along the way, and so many people have said sport is a great background for business. It also makes you a good team member.' (If anyone can take criticism it's Kelly. One of her coaches famously called her a 'wimp' – immediately after winning bronze at the 2004 Olympics – and used to make her do 'wobble tests' on her bottom.)

But you don't have to have played sport at a high level for the EY effect to have an impact. Mumsnet CEO Justine Roberts was sports-mad as a kid, playing in the back garden with her brothers, and still follows her beloved Liverpool FC today. She enjoyed a spell as a sports journalist writing for national newspapers before deciding to carve out a more family-friendly career and set up Mumsnet. The forum is now the biggest discussion site for parents in the UK, and is said to have so much influence that gaining the support of Mumsnetters can win you the general election. The Mumsnet working pattern is exemplary in its design and means that parents can easily be employed across flexible hours. So far, so unsporty. Four children later, and Justine says her interest in sport has massively influenced her career. 'It's helped me hugely,' she says now, 'it's helped in male-dominated environments – it's a great icebreaker talking about sport because you're never stuck for anything to say – but it's also exposed me to how to deal with competition, and how to work in a team. Being in a leadership role, it's no good having one or two high-flyers going off and being brilliant, you need to pull the team along together and that's a very sporting scenario.' Scattered across sport are many more examples – from the female footballer Claire Rafferty, who combines a career as a city analyst at Deutsche Bank with playing left back for Chelsea and England, to qualified lawyer and England striker Eniola Aluko, or Britain's greatest female rower, Katherine Grainger, who also has a PhD in criminal law and homicide.

Out in the real world, though, how many women are there like Kelly, Michelle, Justine, Eniola, Claire or Katherine? Hardly any of my schoolfriends played sport at a serious level. Of the ones who did, most had quit by the time puberty hit. And thirty years on, with PE so low on the list of priorities for schoolchildren, particularly girls, that pattern is not likely to change anytime soon. Do the people in charge of the national curriculum even know that sport can positively affect a woman's future career prospects? Do they ever speak to the Department for Work and Pensions? Do they have a joined-up approach? Because all the rhetoric around engaging young girls in physical activity and 'never mind if it's Zumba rather than, say, cricket' doesn't really cut the mustard. We don't know if Zumba is going to make you more competitive, and EY's research doesn't cover yoga, or Pilates, or aerobics. Of course there's an argument to say that all of those things could potentially offer women similar leadership and workplace skills based around commitment, discipline and hard work. But if it's not the same, and if we're not getting any closer to generating a female workforce with a grounding in sport, then what on earth can we do about it?

For a start, sport needs to be taken more seriously as a platform for creating strong, ambitious and independent-minded young women. Tanni Grey-Thompson thinks sport should have its own government department, away from the 'culture and media' bit, with a minister apiece for sport and physical activity. That's because, despite being hugely influential and potentially life-changing, sport is still seen as a bit of a joke; within newspapers the sports desk is often referred to as 'the toy department'. But sport, particularly for women, has always been so much more than that. It's revolutionary, empowering, radical, and political. It's at the front line of change, and if we want the workplace to change for women – from equal pay to maternity rights – we cannot afford to ignore sport's role here.

Think of the one moment the recent *Suffragette* film would not have considered excluding from its narrative: the story of Emily Davison who slipped underneath the barrier at Epsom and into the path of the king's horse on Derby day in 1913. Emily was an experienced militant activist; she knew what a powerful platform this sporting event was – attended by royalty, high society, journalists and film crews. Her death, captured on camera, remains one of the most enduring images in history of women's struggle for equality. Time and again the suffragettes used sport to raise the profile of their cause, from replacing the flags at King George's own private golf course at Balmoral with suffragette colours and handwritten slogans demanding votes for women, to attacking the then prime minister, Herbert Asquith, as he played a round of golf while on holiday at Elgin. All around the country golf courses were targeted, chemicals poured onto the turf or sections of the greens dug out to spell the slogans: 'Justice before sport' and 'Votes for women'. Cricket pavilions and boathouses were set alight, bowls clubs and grandstands at Crystal Palace and Blackburn's grounds were also attacked. There was even an attempt to burn down Wimbledon, home of the All England Lawn Tennis Association. Why? As the periodical *American Golfer* pointed out at the time, golf was already a popular 'ladies' sport', so wasn't the movement counterproductive to the rights of their own sex? The suffragettes thought not, and Emmeline Pankhurst publicly encouraged these acts for the disruption they caused to what was often seen as the inner sanctum of male bonding and recreation.

In some ways, not much has changed. I have a friend who works in finance. Her boss is middle-aged and keeps a small logbook on his desk. In it he notes down the scores of the young men in the office who play squash. He likes to keep track of who is winning and who is losing. He doesn't play himself, or go to watch them; it is simply an interest maintained from afar. It's his way of assessing the young bucks in the office. A creepy kind of machismo, marvelling over the athletic and competitive abilities of junior male staff, running his eye over future candidates for promotion. Or there's another friend, a TV producer, who remarks, 'It never ceases to amaze me how every time I ask two guys in TV how they know each other, the answer I get is always football. They play football together, or they are into online gaming together.'

Without doubt, sport's influence over the workplace is as ubiquitous as the office tea break. Whether it's sweepstakes during the World Cup, or women being invited to act as 'cheer-leaders' at office football matches (as a male colleague quipped to another friend of mine, 'FA rules do state that women and men cannot engage on the same field of play . . .'), sport has had a place at work for decades.

Take the example of the Bank of England's annual sports day, also known as Governor's Day, which takes place every July at the plush grounds of the Bank of England Sports Club, Roe-hampton. It is the biggest career-networking opportunity in the bank's social calendar, when the Governor and his most senior staff turn out to mingle with the minions. High-profile sports stars are recruited to hand out prizes, and even to play against the staff. It is billed as an 'inclusive' and 'family-friendly' event, with a funfair and food tents, a day at which spouses and children are welcome. So far so jolly, but flick through media reports and the focus seems to be on the all-male cricket and football matches taking place between male staff, plus a sprinkling of male sporting celebrities. At former Governor Sir Mervyn King's farewell sports day in 2013, for example, there was an all-male cricket match and a star-studded five-a-side game between Sir Merv and a selection of the 1982 European Cup-winning Aston Villa players. Turns out Merv was a big Villa fan and fancied playing against his heroes, as did his grandson and some of his colleagues. 'So what happens if you're female and work at the Bank of England?' a friend of mine asked one of the employees. 'Well, you just come along and watch from the side,' she replied.

Some might say this is no surprise for a 320-year-old institution in which senior staff are still attended to by doormen in pink tailcoats and top hats. Or that, at the height of the economic recession in 2009, the Bank advised female employees how not to dress like a prostitute. In case you're wondering, apparently ankle chains should be avoided at all costs, but high heels and lipstick are essential. I'm *so* glad they were thinking about these things. Imagine trying to tackle the financial crisis without the right shoes on.

Not wanting to judge without having sampled the sports day myself, I put in a request to attend Governor's Day. Sadly they have a strict no-media rule, but the press officer did assure me that things have changed significantly since the arrival of Governor Mark Carney in 2013. For one thing, Carney has abolished the game of cricket as the centrepiece of the day, instead preferring rounders and football as examples of more 'inclusive' sports. While traditionalists were up in arms over the decision, many say that Carney's modernizing of such an archaic event is symptomatic of a trend happening across the financial sector.

A similar shift – from traditional sport to the sport of the masses – had an effect on politics in the 1990s, in the form of football. Tony Blair and New Labour's ascent to power coincided with a period of laddism that had at its heart the re-popularization of football – from the launch of the Premier League to Nick Hornby's novel *Fever Pitch* and England hosting the Euros and obsessing over Gazza. It was a period I remember well as a seventeen-year-old, as I perched on the kitchen counter on a hot June day, listening intently to BBC 5 Live on a tiny radio, praying that the Czech Republic would beat Germany in the final. They didn't. It was a seminal summer for me in terms of my relationship to sport. After seventeen years of never quite fitting in with the rest of the population – as part of an immigrant hippy family with bookshelves full of Jung and Milan Kundera, living in a council flat, eating alfalfa sprout sandwiches, and not knowing what a Yorkshire pudding was – finally I was hitting the mainstream. And it was all thanks to football. Football was the common language that could unite us all, across fashion divides, ethnicity, religion and even gender. And I was buying in. Massively. At the time my dad said he couldn't understand why girls would be interested in watching men play football, a comment he later apologized for. But my dad was out of touch with the mood of the nation. England was going football crazy. The 'Three Lions' (Football's Coming Home) anthem gave us all a way to be patriotic without being parochial. This wasn't about ugly nationalism. In its new guise, football was more acceptable than ever, and influencing some of the most unlikely institutions.

That change in football's status and influence cannot be underestimated. And so it was that an electorate watched as Tony Blair played head tennis with then Newcastle manager Kevin Keegan at the 1995 Labour Party conference, and decided that this was the man to lead the nation. Blair even took advice from former Manchester United manager Sir Alex Ferguson on leadership. ('What would you do if your best player won't do what you want him to and just does his own thing?' Blair recalls asking, in his memoirs. 'Chuck him out of the team,' was Ferguson's alleged reply.) When Blair and Brown wanted to show a united front following rumours of ongoing disagreements, they arranged a photo opportunity in which both men sat watching football on the TV and drinking beer. The whole party was so steeped in football that if you wanted to get ahead, you needed to be on the bandwagon.

How did this new dynamic affect women in the political world? In 2008 the *Financial Times*'s political editor George Parker wrote an eye-opening article titled 'Power Games', charting football's role in politics. His assertion, that football made the Labour Party something akin to a Sunday league team outing, is both fascinating and frightening. What if you weren't a football fan? How were you supposed to get on? 'Football has been a thread throughout Labour's decade in power,' he wrote. 'It greases the wheels of politics; it is a networking tool; it is a political message.' Parker described how even under the leadership of Gordon Brown – a passionate Raith Rovers fan – football was central to working processes. 'Brown regularly mapped out economic policy over football and pizza in the Grosvenor House Hotel apartment of Geoffrey Robinson, a fellow Treasury minister and football fanatic,' he wrote.[13] He details how football came to exert such an influence on the corridors of power in Westminster that civil servants and journalists attempted to ingratiate themselves by swotting up on the football scores from the weekend just so that they could make small talk with the ministers come Monday morning.

Parker's specific focus was a team made up of New Labour employees, called 'Demon Eyes' (a reference to the Tories' controversial general election poster of 1997 in which Blair was depicted with devilish red eyes). In its football incarnation, Demon Eyes was a bunch of middle-class Islingtonians who trained on Highbury Fields and competed in the tough Thames League (twice winning promotion, and a Division One title in 2001). 'We had a reputation as a fairly unpleasant team to play against,' recalls Andy Burnham, now shadow home secretary. 'We all backed each other up quite a lot. It could get quite fruity.' One of Blair's aides is alleged to have got involved in a punch-up, and Demon Eyes even had their own war cry: 'Winners!' they would yell. The list of names involved in that team reads like a *Who's Who* of politics: from Burnham to James Purnell, Ed Balls to David Miliband.

It all sounds distinctly laddish, a theme that didn't escape some women at the time. In 1998, Helen Wilkinson, co-founder of the Blairite think tank Demos, publicly denounced the Labour government's 'new lad culture' in a column for the *New Statesman*. She revealed how brainstorming sessions at Chequers regularly ended up with advisers playing five-a-side football on the lawns. 'This "new lad culture" seems harmless enough and is justified in terms of team bonding,' she said. 'The problem is that team bonding too readily turns to male bonding. The old boys' network may have progressed from golf to football, but the fundamental rules are the same.'

Unless, of course, you were a woman daring enough to join them – like Jo Gibbons. A long-time Labour staffer, who went on to work for Tony Blair for many years, Gibbons is now a board member of Women in Sport. She played on the women's Number 10 Downing Street team ('we only ever had one fixture, against Buckingham Palace women's team, and they were terrifying, all ex-RAF and military'), but she also forced herself to join in with the Sunday morning kickarounds on Highbury

Fields that many of the Demon Eyes team players took part in, one of a very few women who did.

Despite no background in playing football – which was banned for girls when she was growing up – Jo was passionate about the game. Demon Eyes was an all men's team of course, but in those Sunday morning kickabouts with influential Labour Party rising stars she saw football as an obvious way of further-ing her career. 'I immediately recognized the opportunities involved,' she says now. 'Through football I built relationships, it was part of my personal networking experience, no doubt about it. A female friend of mine was also a Labour Party press officer but her relationships weren't as strong as mine, I'm sure that's because of football.' I can't help but admire her gutsiness in joining the team, and the strong career plan she had in the back of her mind even then. Jo describes an era in which politics was 'alpha male' and populated by 'hard-drinking, football-loving blokes'. If you wanted to get on, you did well to fit in. Her sister, formerly a marketing executive, had a similar experi-ence in her industry – learning to play golf in order to take out clients and strengthen her relationships. So is this the takeaway message for women in the twenty-first century?

Fiona Hathorn, Managing Director of Women on Boards in the UK, an organization pushing to change the gender balance across some of the most powerful boardrooms in the country, echoes Jo's experiences. Fiona learned about sport and business the hard way. As a fund manager in the 1990s she noticed that her male colleagues were forever going on golf or shooting days, or spending corporate time watching Formula One or football or Wimbledon. Although Fiona didn't come from a sporty family, a word in her ear from her female boss encouraged her to get to grips with the basics. 'My boss told me I must make time to network because relationships are key to speaking to the right stockbrokers and getting the best information first. It was all who you knew, and did they call you first. She said: you need to get out there.' So Fiona learned to play golf, and to shoot, and to do just about anything involving sport. Because sport, she says, is the preferred means of business networking. And networking in business is the gospel.

According to leadership business guru Herminia Ibarra, there are three main types of network to know about.

1) Operational: that's the people around you in your workplace. 'Women are normally very good at those relationships,' says Fiona, 'although not usually outside their own department. And that's exactly where you need to network in order to get up the ladder.'

2) Personal: that could be anything from your social circle, to how you interact when picking the kids up from school. Fiona believes that men naturally champion their achievements in their social circles, talking about work at the school gate, at football, on a night out with friends. 'It's much harder for women,' says Fiona. 'For example, when I'd pick my kids up from school I had to choose between making friends with the other mums at the school gate, or making a beeline for the dad who works at Deutsche Bank so I can network with him. How judged will I be? You'd never see a guy worrying about that. And that's very stereotypical about the way we are still bringing girls up – to please.'

3) Strategic: which is all about conferences and corporate days out. 'Sport plays a big part in these,' says Fiona. 'If you're in the office and your team is obsessed with cricket and you don't know anything about cricket you're out of the group, your relationships possibly aren't going to be as strong. Those people who tend to do well blur the work–life boundaries.'

That's because business is essentially far more about personal relationships than we like to believe. Think of *The Wolf of Wall Street*, in which Jordan Belfort assembles a team of complete losers to run what ends up being a multimillion-dollar company. But those losers are not any old losers, they're his friends. Now we all like to accept that the best people for the job get the job. Or that headhunting is all about searching out expertise. But we *know* that's not always the case. And that's because we're human beings. We like personal connections. We like things to laugh about together, we like to feel comfortable in each other's company.

Fiona believes that sharing sports experiences can break down barriers to personal connection, and that's why they're so valued in the business sector. 'It's all the funny incidents that happen that create close relationships. Like one time I went karting, and I'm only small. They didn't have a boiler suit for a woman so I was put in a huge outfit for a big guy. I had to roll the sleeves up and the legs up and everyone was just killing themselves laughing from looking at me. But I came second in the go-karting because I'm very light, and I drive very aggressively, braking and accelerating at the same time. And months later I'd be travelling the Asian markets and bump into people who would say, "Oh! Do you remember that stupid suit! That was so funny!" and we'd laugh about it together. And what I've seen is people being given job offers through those relationships.'

Listening to Fiona and Jo, I can't help but feel my heart sink, just a little. I am full of admiration for their get up and go, I'm just not sure I could ever emulate it. Are we saying this is the only solution? Learn to play golf? Shoot? Be one of the boys? It could all start to feel a bit forced. Like those US websites designed to help women talk sport around the nation's water coolers – *Heels & Helmets: Ladies, Get in the Game and Win!* or *Talk Sports Like a Pro: 99 Secrets to Becoming a Sports Goddess.* Maybe these initiatives have worked wonders for some women's careers, but if I'm honest I find them a bit weird. Like 'fake it till you make it' guides on how to bag a boyfriend. Can't we just be ourselves?

Fiona sympathizes. 'A Muslim woman said the same thing to me after a presentation I did recently. She said, "Do you know, I feel really depressed now. I knew I was stuffed because I was female and a minority, I'm further stuffed because I'm Muslim and I wear a hijab, and now I'm doubly stuffed because I don't like sport. I haven't got a frickin' chance." I thought that was a really great thing she said, because it's up to great leaders to ensure they're thinking about the diversity of their client base. Your spending should reflect your existing client base but also what your client base hopes to be like in ten years' time.'

Currently that's just not happening enough. Fiona talks about a day out at Lord's Cricket Ground recently where she counted twenty-seven corporate boxes, approximately twenty people per box, and just two women. 'It's in those boxes that the networking happens, people getting slightly tipsy, having a laugh. But men naturally invite other men; they need to start inviting women and women need to start forcing themselves to go.' But what if you don't like sport? You're not familiar with cricket? You're worried about being quizzed on batting averages? 'In all honesty, half of them aren't really watching the sport anyway; they're getting drunk, eating lunch and bonding. I don't like F1 but I still loved the day out, it was fabulous. You've got to view networking as, "I'm going to meet interesting people," not, "Oh my God, I don't want to go." You've got to have a plan: "Right, I'll do two conferences a year and four away days." You can't do all of it, but make sure you're there for some of it.'

Sue Unerman, advertising guru and chief strategy officer for MediaCom, tells me the same thing. She doesn't much like sport, and she often turns down corporate invitations to attend sporting events ('I haven't got to where I am today by going to golf days,' she quips). And yet, on her wall, there are yellow Post-it notes about the 'Fosbury Flop' and British cycling guru Dave Brailsford. I don't get it?

'I use sporting analogies at work,' explains Sue, a rare example of a woman at the top of her field who has spent many years working part-time. 'I've been doing it for fifteen years because you get immediate understanding, particularly from men. There's nothing more effective than a football analogy. You could spend hours researching how to sell an idea with statistics and charts, or you could say, "who do we want to beat, Barcelona or Fulham?" and that will get heads nodding in a meeting. I'm speaking their language.' Because she doesn't watch sport Sue gets her analogies from her partner, Mark, a huge West Ham fan. She explains the situation at work, and asks him for a comparable example from the world of sport. The analogies she gives me are so illuminating that I find myself nodding and grinning, even though I know absolutely nothing about advertising, multimillion-pound billings, or how to make a profit in business. When she talks sport, I – a business ignoramus – actually understand what she's on about. What's more, the process feels enjoyable.

'I remember I had one client who was incredibly analytical. He obsessed over his style of thinking and was reluctant to try anything else. But I wanted him to throw that approach out for the day, so in our meeting I put up a picture of Barcelona losing to Chelsea in the Champions League semi-final in 2012. I said that at that moment, losing to Chelsea at the Nou Camp, Barcelona fans the world over were screaming at their TVs, "just put it in the mixer!" I didn't actually know what that meant, but Mark had explained to me that Barcelona were famous for their analytical style of play, and that sometimes stymies the element of surprise that wins you the Champions League semi-final. The thing is that people really love that you're using language they understand, instead of advertising jargon. I also have a Tiger Woods one which is brilliantly effective. It deals with the debate about whether companies should invest in innovation, or focus on profits. I say, "So if Tiger Woods earns 10 per cent of his salary from golf competitions, and 90 per cent of his income from sponsorship, where should he invest his hours?" That one's even more pertinent since his fall from grace . . .'

Sue was put off sport at an early age by a golf-obsessed grandmother ('she'd make me caddy for her every weekend at the golf club in Potters Bar', one of the first set up specifically for the Jewish community who weren't allowed in clubs elsewhere) and by always being last pick for teams at school. 'My experience of sport was to fail,' she says. Sue believes it had a lasting impact on her ability to work within a group. 'I didn't understand about teams early on in my career. I was a perfectionist and focused on how great my work was. But I learned, and what I discovered was that I was so competitive it was just all being sublimated. I eventually learned to put my effort into getting the team to win. And the pleasure of doing that together is incredible, while the comfort of failing together is immense. I'm only sorry I didn't learn it at school. Teamwork in sport is about understanding that it doesn't matter how lovely someone is; if they drop the baton they've let you down. Similarly you shouldn't care if someone is an arsehole so long as they deliver in their role. It's the neutrality of sport, it's all about the performance.'

I can relate to what Sue is saying because it has taken me years to embrace being part of a team. As a child at school I hated it; I'd inwardly groan when we had to work in groups, I didn't know how to make the most of the different skill sets around the table and I would withdraw and let others make the decisions. Like Sue, I was continually drawn to personalities over practicalities. If I liked someone I wanted to work with them, regardless of whether they were great or useless at the task they were given. Twenty-five years down the line and I've finally learned to love – and understand – teamwork. With Women in Football, the industry networking organization that I chair, I feel so proud of our collective achievements. I get a thrill seeing others excel in their strengths, which in turn makes us all stronger. But I can't help wondering if I could have learned all this a long time ago and saved myself a lot of internal angst and inefficient working. And, more to the point, how are we going to ensure the next generation of young women don't fall into the same trap?

Even if the government does suddenly bring in a raft of

changes to school sport that ensures my daughter won't miss out on a sporting skill set, what about the millions of women for whom it is already too late? Do they really have to learn to shoot and play golf? Fake it to make it? Are cricket, football – even paintball – the only options to help with team bonding and productivity? Isn't there another way to reap the benefits of sport in the workplace, without alienating those who have never played – or enjoyed playing – sport before? I know I've been guilty of routinely turning down pretty much every sporting opportunity that's ever come my way in my career, except for maybe tenpin bowling at an office Christmas party. That's where Georgie Bullen's story comes in. The GB captain for Goalball, a Paralympic sport for blind and visually impaired teams, she takes her sport into workplaces across the country, blindfolding employees and getting them to try relay races and Goalball drills. 'It's much more effective than falling backwards into your colleagues' arms,' says Georgie, who believes that depriving employees of one of their key senses – sight – teaches people how to communicate better and, ultimately, trust each other.[14]

If I'm honest, when I hear about sportspeople setting up businesses to complement their sporting careers I tend to feel a bit sceptical. They'll put their name to a swim club, a nutrition plan or sports product, and it can all feel a bit half-hearted, something to help the cash flow. Georgie's story is very different. She's only twenty-one and she's extraordinary. Her business, supported by the Prince's Trust and the Royal National Institute for the Blind, is genuinely helpful to workplaces; it also creates awareness of visual impairment in a playful way as employees get to try out simulation spectacles recreating varying degrees of blindness. But Georgie doesn't shy away from some of the hard-hitting facts about life with a visual impairment in the UK, either. I was gobsmacked when she told me that two-thirds of working-age blind and VI people in this country are un-employed. She relays the story of her GB teammate's blind husband. 'He's been job-hunting for years; he can't get anything. He's got a degree, he's very smart. It's not through lack of trying. He started out wanting to use his degree, but ended up applying for any admin job he could find. I really want to help that. I went to mainstream schools and all I needed to be included was to make sure worksheets were enlarged type.'

Through Paralympic sport Georgie found life. It's as simple as that. At her mainstream school she was sidelined in PE les-sons, the teachers told her she was no good, and she was always the last in the line when it came to picking teams. This was a pretty confusing state of affairs for a girl who grew up playing sport with her brothers in the back garden and saw it as a normal thing to do. Georgie had wanted to study PE for GCSE, but was discouraged by her teachers who felt she wouldn't be able to cope. Little did they know that she would go on to captain her country at the greatest sporting event the UK has ever host-ed, London 2012. You have to wonder how many other, less determined, kids were left behind because they did not receive the encouragement or opportunity to take part in sport. I know many adult women who often reflect, with genuine curiosity, on how talented they might have been at sport – had they only been given a proper chance.

Georgie's story makes me angry. The upshot, of course, is that she found Paralympic sport and, surrounded by other ath-letes with visual impairments, she instantly discovered a support network of friends who could laugh and rage about all the crazy things they have in common through their disability. Like being chased down the street by an angry stranger convinced that they were in pursuit of someone who had stolen a guide dog. 'People just don't understand visual impairment, they think you're either blind or you're fully sighted. A lot of people struggle to understand that disability is anything other than being in a wheelchair.' Sometimes it's the everyday comments that get to her. 'Like when people realize you're visually impaired and they say, "Oh, that's a such a shame because you're so pretty."' Georgie laughs. I am speechless.

What's so clever about Georgie's business is how it uses Paralympic sport to teach able-bodied people something important, to improve their capacity in their everyday jobs. This is such a significant inversion of the usual narrative where mainstream society helps Paralympic sport, or disabled people in general, prompted by some sort of moral obligation. Instead, Georgie's scheme is about what disability can teach the rest of us. And how incredibly powerful those lessons can be. Because while the Paralympics are all good, the English Federation of Disability Sport says two-thirds of disabled people don't want to take part in segregated sport; they want to join in with everyone else. And even for those interested in pursuing an elite career in sport, the Paralympics represent only a small section of the disabled community because of the limited number of classifications available. The world is so set up for able-bodied people that, from the workplace to our discussions around health, we routinely exclude anyone with a disability.

And what if you're actively banned from taking part in sport in your workplace? It sounds extreme, but that's the situation that sports minister Tracey Crouch found herself in as an up-and-coming MP. We meet in her offices, opposite Parliament Square. She is several months pregnant but hardly shows, her blouse neatly tucked into a pencil skirt, while I negotiate my own enormous-feeling pregnancy bump to reach for a mug of tea. Astonishingly, she is the first Tory minister ever to take maternity leave.

Tracey grew up playing every sport under the sun, even when teachers in the playground told her not to. 'You're not allowed to play,' they'd say, 'go and do something else.' She coached a girls' football team for nine years alongside her political career, and follows pretty much every other sport. She's a rare example of a sports minister who can take on the media's dreaded inauguration sports quiz without her advisors breaking into a sweat.

I first heard about Tracey when she complained of being excluded from the parliamentary football team, in 2011. I tentatively ask about it now, wondering if since she has become the sports minister she would prefer not to go over old ground. But her response and feeling on the matter seem as strong as ever.

'By the time I got elected in 2010 the FA were running the team and felt it was necessary to adhere to all FA rules, and of course they ban mixed football over a certain age. I was unable to play for any team that the FA coordinated. That meant the parliamentary team but also the teams that are put out at party conference. It's all to do with the referee and insurance. Although many of the professional referees I've spoken to have said they'd be happy to do it,' she adds. At the Conservative Party conference the team decided to allow Tracey to play, and forfeited the FA's financial assistance with kit and referees. That's a heavy burden to carry for one player. It seems a ridiculous state of affairs, particularly now that Tracey is sports minister. Surely the FA cannot continue to stick to their archaic stance and deny the minister a place on the team? There must be a solution to this? 'I don't think there is one unless the FA is more flexible in its attitude to running a parliamentary football team,' sighs Tracey. 'The way it's run can be taken a bit too seriously. The players on the team say I'd be very welcome to take part. When you've got people visiting parliament there will be ladies who want to come along and play. But I think the FA probably just need to take themselves a little bit less seriously on this issue. And until they do that there's no way forward.' She folds her arms in her lap, but I am irate. 'But Tracey, you are the sports minister! This is insane!' I say. 'Yeah,' says Tracey, 'I'll just have to withdraw all their funding or something . . .' she jokes. Tracey says she agrees that sport is an important part of networking and the workplace and that she doesn't feel women should have to miss out on it. 'I don't feel I've personally missed out on networking or engagement with my colleagues, but I think people should always have the opportunity to participate in a sport if they want to.'

So what is she doing about the next generation? Tracey is far more positive about the future than I am, reflecting on how opportunities for young women have improved since she was a girl. I suppose it is the job of a politician to be optimistic; I only wish there was closer collaboration between the various government departments. As Tracey says, 'There's always room for improvement [in school sport] but it's not within my department's scope to monitor it . . .' Thankfully, Tracey's initiative of a new sports strategy focuses heavily on grass roots, and ropes in multiple departments to consult. 'We are looking at all age groups; we know that older people who are physically active are going to be less of a drain on the NHS because physical activity reduces loneliness and isolation, so it's good for people to be involved.' Best of all, the 2016 strategy targets children from five years old and upwards. This is huge and welcome progress, particularly considering that the old approach only sought to encourage young people into sport once they had turned fourteen.

And while she's a total sports nut, Tracey says she has learned to love Zumba, which makes me warm to her. 'I was a real sceptic to start with,' she says, 'not least because I have no coordination for dancing, but the Zumba class I used to go to was held in a village hall where the instructor turned off the lights and only illuminated the stage, so it didn't matter if I was the person at the back that looked like a muppet because no one could see you. I'd come away sweating more at Zumba than I ever did at football. And you can do it by yourself.'

From doing Zumba in semi-darkness, to the ever-evolving workplace. A coffee with EY Head of Sponsorship Tom Kingsley proves to be a refreshing conversation as he talks about rounds of golf being replaced by walking lunch meetings, or cycle rides up Box Hill. He says much of this is down to companies coming under pressure to be more inclusive – and with women rising through the ranks there are new interests to embrace. This, in turn, could have an important knock-on effect for women's sport – a point that Fiona highlights. If golf tournaments now feel stuffy and ubiquitous, then how about sponsoring women's rugby, or rowing, or football? Female staff members are more likely to be interested in joining a sporting environment if women are the focus, and it has huge corporate social responsibility benefits for the company at a time when 'femvertising' is all the rage in the commercial sector.

But the change isn't just about women. It's also about men. One of the best things Tom tells me is that, with two young children at home, he doesn't want to miss out on family time because of corporate networking responsibilities. So if he's invited to a Champions League game midweek, he'd rather be at home, get the kids to bed, then pop downstairs and watch it on the telly. Or if it's a sporting event at the weekend, he wants to make sure it doesn't eat into family time – so he'll ask, can he bring his wife? Or his two boys? His family are Liverpool supporters and he says he'll always ask if he can bring his sons with him to a game. He'll swap the corporate hospitality for regular tickets, and then nip upstairs to the box at half-time for a business coffee. He's aware that the older generation might not be comfortable with all this, but as a dad with young kids he's got a strong sense of what kind of environment he wants to work in, and how it can be better for everybody.

As mum to a young daughter, I find Tom's anecdotes really cheer my heart. This is the modern dad at work. And I want there to be more of them. I remember after I had my daughter a male colleague brought his baby to work in a sling one day. There was widespread comment on this phenomenon, and discussion of whether it should be seen as a brilliant act from a liberated man, or yet more proof that men can get away with things that women wouldn't dare to. '*You* wouldn't have brought a baby to a press conference,' one of my colleagues said, 'because if you had, well, just think of the furore.'

The comment reminded me of that old Chris Rock sketch about men getting credit for things they should be doing anyway. Men who say, 'I take care of my kids.' 'Yeah,' Chris Rock retorts, 'you're supposed to, you dumb motherfucker!' That culture makes a lot of women angry. Why should men be praised for doing the things that many mothers do every single day, such as looking after their kids? But while I understand that frustration, I also think there's something important about the role that fathers can play in creating change for everyone. And what better place to do that than at work? Perhaps we should thank those individuals for leading the way.

I certainly think that what Tom is describing is part of a bigger trend away from the traditional way of working, towards workplace relationships that are more human. But no less sporty. Over the summer a lawyer friend invited me to join a networking sports league for men and women. Usually that sort of thing sends me running. But what was so clever about this initiative is that she chose sports that most people were unlikely to be well practised in – reaffirming the importance of Georgie's concept in creating a level playing field to make sport as inclusive as possible. Mixed teams took on the challenges, guided by an expert who provided a quick masterclass at the start of each event, including softball, rounders, and my personal favourite: lawn bowls.

If anything, with the rising number of remote workers and increased online communication replacing face-to-face meetings, the work environment needs the human touch more than ever. And as we face issues of burnout and stress and email overload, we need employees to be fitter and healthier, to take mental breaks, to get away from their screens. Sport and exercise are a brilliant way to achieve this. A recent article in *Forbes* magazine boasted about the six ways that exercise boosts brain productivity – including improved blood flow to the brain for around two to three hours after being active, releasing endorphins which help the brain to prioritize and focus on tasks, and also an improvement in memory. Kathrine Switzer and her 1970s ode to the marathon's capacity to stimulate intellectual thought are clearly still relevant today in this modern trend where sport, exercise and the workplace are all moving closer together.

Over a decade ago, starting out as a young sports journalist, I was part of the early days of this movement. Along with another young female writer, I signed up to take lunchtime yoga classes at work. The teacher was pretty hardcore about his vinyasas, and I'll never forget giggling our heads off about one of his favourite sequences which involved putting your 'heel in your anus'. But the bond we formed in those sessions was much more than learning some crazy yoga moves. Ultimately, putting our heel in our anus enabled us to become a vital support for each other in a very male-dominated sector. I'm not sure either of us would have survived without the other.

Across the workplace more and more organizations are being converted to this way of thinking. Team bonding, greater concentration at work, healthier staff meaning less sick days – from the record companies who hire in Pilates teachers to instruct employees in their lunch breaks, and the city workers heading off to the boxing gym together each morning, to the personal trainers heading into office blocks with kettlebells each day, and the phone companies setting up table-tennis tables for 'creative thinking'.

The great thing is, you don't need to be in an office doing sport to feel some of these benefits. Getting your brain going in the morning could be as simple as ditching the car on the school run. Or exchanging your stress-filled daily commute to work by public transport for a forty-minute walk through the city. The health apps on our phones now automatically measure how far we walk each day, down to how many flights of stairs we climb, as even the smallest bit of physical activity sends our brains into appreciative serotonin-fuelled ecstasy. Best of all, exercise makes us feel as though we have accomplished something important before we even sit down to face that dreaded tax return, or endless piles of marking. It gives us that lift to help us get on with the day. With our jobs becoming more sedentary but more mentally demanding than ever, getting away from our desks, cash registers, vehicles and computers is essential. And it works at any time of day. The lunchtime run lifts our energy for the rest of the afternoon, while the after-work dip in the river Thames – taking advantage of the wild swimming craze – is pure magic, the water lapping at your torso as the stress of the day slowly recedes. Ultimately, whether it's to get ahead in our career, or just to help us stay sane, make no mistake about it: sport and exercise is our lifeline to surviving the twenty-first-century workplace.

Sport and taboos

We should have started talking about periods in sport years ago. The sportswomen were happy to oblige, dropping the hints. Why didn't we pick up the baton and run with it? Instead there was just this enormous elephant in the room, ignored by journalists, coaches, medics, sports scientists and sports governing bodies.

Serena Williams was one of the first to break the taboo back in 2005 when she revealed that she suffered from menstrual migraines. In the UK the story hardly got a mention; in the US there was more coverage but it wasn't headline news. Jelena Jankovic then blamed 'women's problems' for her third-round defeat at Wimbledon in 2009. The way the press responded to the former world number one was extraordinary. Despite Jelena expressing concern that she might have needed an ambulance because she felt so dizzy and unwell, journalists accused her of being a drama queen. 'One year it is parking lots and helicopters; the next year it is "women's problems",' wrote one journalist in the *Telegraph*, as though the two were interchangeable.[15]

When it comes to period pains, there's nothing like telling a woman she's just being melodramatic. 'Some doctors tell you it's mental,' agreed Serena. 'One of my doctors actually told me that. "You have to get over it. There's nothing really wrong with you. You just think it is when it gets to be that time of the month." I was thinking, "I've got to be more mentally tough."' When she finally got a proper diagnosis it turned out that she was suffering from menstrual migraines, a debilitating chronic condition for which she now takes medication. 'I know it doesn't look like it affected my tennis,' said Serena, who at that point had already won seven Grand Slam titles. 'But especially in the sun, playing with a migraine makes it worse. In Australia it's not that easy. I remember playing Martina Hingis in Sydney, and I was just out of it. You want to just crawl under your bed and stay there,' she added. 'I want to tell women my story, to let them know there is hope and they should seek help.'[16]

A decade on, and society has finally begun to catch up. At the start of 2015 two little words blew open a brave new world for women and menstruation. 'Girl things', said British tennis player Heather Watson after she was knocked out of the Australian Open, citing dizziness, nausea and low energy levels so bad she was forced to call a doctor towards the end of the first set.

Thankfully, this time around the press responded in a completely different way, and an avalanche of coverage about menstruation suddenly found its way into the mainstream media, with sports desks frantically calling every female athlete in their contacts book and asking them to talk about *that time of the month*. For women it was pretty bizarre; after all, periods are not a new development. It still took a little adjustment for some, however. I remember a colleague asking her editor if she could cover the subject and he said he'd need to check that their readers were 'ready for it'.

Now that we could openly talk about periods, we learned just how much sportswomen had been silently putting up with for years. From Wimbledon's archaic insistence that all players must wear white and only take one toilet break per set, regardless of how long that set lasts, to the embarrassment of providing urine samples for drugs testers at that time of the month – never mind the pain, inconvenience, injury issues and discomfort. The conversation certainly forced me to reassess the famous incident of French tennis star Tatiana Golovin and her 'saucy red knickers', as the tabloids breathlessly described them. They looked more like sports shorts, and I'm now wondering if she wore them because she was on her period. I do hope so, because the irony of Fleet Street getting so hot under the collar about some 'French knickers', when they were just period pants, is too funny. Thankfully, in amongst all the horror stories there are also some examples of best practice – such as GB women's hockey, where teammates frequently talk about their periods, while their medical department track their monthly cycles. Unfortunately those examples are all too few and far between.

But if Heather Watson opened the door to talking about menstruation in sport, then Kiran Gandhi, a former drummer with MIA, blasted it off its hinges when she decided to run the 2015 London Marathon without sanitary protection. Kiran had trained for a year leading up to the event, but when her period started the night before the race she had a radical idea. She would run the marathon and free-bleed. It would be a show of support for all the women in the world who cannot afford sanitary protection. And it would do away with the dilemma of whether to struggle for 26.2 miles with a tampon in, or face the chafing hell of sanitary towels.

'I thought, if there's one person society won't fuck with, it's a marathon runner,' she later wrote on her blog. 'If there's one way to transcend oppression, it's to run a marathon in whatever way you want. On the marathon course, sexism can be beaten. Where the stigma of a woman's period is irrelevant, and we can re-write the rules as we choose. Where a woman's comfort supersedes that of the observer. I ran with blood dripping down my legs for sisters who don't have access to tampons and sisters who, despite cramping and pain, hide it away and pretend like it doesn't exist. I ran to say, it does exist, and we overcome it every day. The marathon was radical and absurd and bloody in ways I couldn't have imagined until the day of the race.'[17]

Kiran found the experience liberating. Her friends ran the entire course alongside her, as a pool of menstrual blood collected in her leggings, while her father and brother greeted her with a warm embrace at the finish line, congratulating her on the $6,000 she had raised for breast cancer. 'It's a radical notion realizing that on a marathon course you don't have to worry about how you look for others.'

The act attracted national media attention. But while the likes of Caitlin Moran hailed her 'punk rock' power, a volley of abusers on social media called her 'disgusting and unhygienic'. Even within the race itself Kiran was approached by other runners sharing their opinion. 'Someone came up behind me making a disgusted face to tell me in a subdued voice that I was on my period . . . I was like . . . wow, I had NO idea!' she wrote on Medium.com.

Ultimately, the disapproval only serves to underline her central point – that women are consistently shamed into hiding their menstrual cycle. While this may be an achievable act for women with average-to-high incomes, the reality is that many women in the world are ostracized from the workplace, from social situations, even from their own family homes while menstruating because of the stigma attached to periods. In India that stigma is captured in the saying, 'don't touch the pickle jar' – when menstruating women are shamed as dirty and impure, banned from the kitchen and places of worship. It's reported that in India one in five girls drop out of school when they start their periods. In 2015 Procter & Gamble won an award for their advert challenging this damaging tradition, and promoting their sanitary protection 'Whisper' (otherwise known as Always). But Kiran writes that just 12 per cent of women in India have access to sanitary pads or tampons; the rest use rags, leaves, even sawdust to stem the flow. To my mind, the Whisper campaign, while admirable to westerners, only further entrenches the idea that disposable sanitary protection is needed for true liberation – as opposed to Kiran's standpoint that menstrual taboos need to be debunked. Meanwhile, in the US forty million women live on the brink of poverty and struggle to meet the cost of a year's supply of sanitary protection – around $70 – a sum not covered by food stamps. In the UK, Kiran's act comes at a timely moment when parliament is debating whether to remove VAT from sanitary protection – a levy that does not currently apply to Jaffa cakes, razors or condoms. In the UK the average amount of money a woman spends on sanitary products is £18,000 across a lifetime. That's almost a year's wages for most women.

But if having a period is troublesome in everyday life, it can be more challenging still for anyone engaged in sport or exercise. One of the most powerful stories to come out of elite sport on this subject was an interview with Paula Radcliffe. The marathon world-record holder revealed that she had warned British Athletics over their use of the drug noresthisterone – which prevents periods during competition – because she said it had caused problems for herself and Jo Pavey in the past. More specifically, she argued, it had caused middle-distance starlet Jessica Judd to fail in the first round of the 2013 World Championships. It opened up a debate about what advice sports governing bodies should be giving athletes around menstruation.

Curious to know more, I spoke to Great Britain's Marilyn Okoro, a promising middle-distance runner whose career had too often been plagued by injury. It was years, however, before anyone suggested there could be a connection between her injuries and her periods. 'I actually didn't think that my period impacted on me at all,' she says, 'but as I got older I've learned more about it. For example my hamstrings and long history of tendinopathy. I started to see a pattern just before I was about to come on – the pain in my left hamstring was just unbearable. I would mention it every now and again to my physios and they would shrug it off. It was only when I was being treated by a female physio, Lily Devine, that I ever had a medical opinion on it. She said, oh, well, that makes perfect sense because all this stuff is happening with your hip movement – your hips are getting wider and it has a direct impact on your hamstring tendon, and she advised me on the things I could do to alleviate that. As I've got older I've realized it affected me a lot.

'Lily was one of the best physios I've ever worked with. She would also know not to put acupuncture needles in me around the time of my period because it would be so painful – normally I can take it but not then. I remember one time she said, "Is it your time of the month? You should always tell me because it's not a good idea. Everything's super sensitive." I've got thick fascia and so it was like torture. But the guys would always be like, "Oh come on, you're just being a wimp," and whack the needles in.'

In a sport like athletics, where half of the athletes are female, I find it desperately disappointing that there are still so few female personnel. Female coaches, in particular, are vastly under-represented. At the 2015 Athletics World Champion-ships, for example, just two out of thirty-nine British athletes' coaches were female: Christine Bowmaker and Carol Williams. Marilyn says she has always steered away from female coaches, choosing men instead. It is a preference I have heard over and over again from female athletes, and one that makes me sad. Where does it come from? Athletes tell me it's just a reflection of the status quo: successful coaches are male, female coaches are – largely – invisible. It reminds me of the video asking young children if Santa could ever be a woman. Apparently not, they say, because she'd 'get lost in the sky' or be too busy having babies. Scarily enough, similar stereotypes persist about female coaches and their ability to be authoritative, or commit to an elite role. It's that age-old dilemma: if you can't see it, you can't be it. But times are changing and, interestingly, Marilyn now wonders how much more open a coach–athlete relationship she might have had with a female coach.

I ask Marilyn if her male doctors or physios ever spoke to her about periods. She says the full extent of the conversation was simply filling in forms with the date of her last cycle, or offering her the delaying pill if she didn't want to be on her period during a major championships. Marilyn always turned the latter option down 'because I feel the pill messes with my hormones'. She says pretty much every athlete she knows who's been offered the contraceptive implant – inserted under the skin in the upper arm – has ended up having it removed because the side effects were so severe. 'The people I spoke to said it made them "crazy" with depression – which is prevalent in sport anyway – anxiousness, heightened irritability, added weight, all of which sounds disastrous to me. I don't need the implant to experience some of those symptoms. I'm not too sure why it was recommended for athletes but it's supposed to be a popular choice because it's tucked away and not invasive.'

Lily aside, did *anyone* in athletics ever speak to Marilyn about her periods? She laughs. 'Obviously track is just so dominated by male coaches, and my coach is great but he does not get it. Things like, "You know that's not an excuse," and then it's the other extreme like, "I've got to go easy on you guys" – like it's some sort of disease,' she says. 'It feels like male coaches just don't know what to do, to be honest. When we go away for champs we have all these booklets and stuff to prepare and there's never anything about that time of the month. The most advice I get is from my nutritionist about diet and how it can help. I get an insatiable appetite craving fried and salty stuff, so I try to eat more greens to counteract that and drink a lot to help with bloating, taking evening primrose oil ten days before it's due, and my supplements and eating smaller portions.' Marilyn says the emotional effects of her period are worse than the physical ones. 'It does make you self-conscious and paranoid, more than normal. I hate it because I feel so bloated I think I look like Michelin Woman, so I worry about stupid things like that my belly will be out [in competition kit], but as long as I don't feel pain then I know I'm feeling worse than I look. You can usually tell if someone is on their period – like if it's someone who usually wears knickers and then wears shorts. I always double up and bring extra stuff in my bag just in case. And make sure my racing uniform colour is friendly.' I ask her if she ever discusses the emotional side of things with her sports psychologist, and she shakes her head. 'No, but I don't know if that's because he's male.' She laughs.

For Kelly Sotherton, the former British heptathlete, the link between periods and injury was always apparent. 'If I had an injury it was often because it was the week before my period and that's why it happened,' she tells me. 'I always felt sluggish ... so we changed my training to be three weeks on and one week off, the rest week would be the week prior to the period because that's when your body's getting ready to have a period and that would always be when I'd get a niggle. That helped a lot towards preventing injury.' Kelly made sure that her coach and the medical team were kept up to date with her periods, though she concedes that not everyone is able to be so open on a subject that many people still see as a taboo. 'I'm a very open person,' says Kelly. 'I wasn't afraid of saying to my coach: this is happening, I'm on my period, I'm a bit sluggish. You have to tell your coach everything or they can't help you. I really had to ensure that my coach knew what was going on. As soon as September came around I'd start planning for next year's championships and changing my periods so they wouldn't clash with the major competitions. I'd plan really far ahead because I wasn't a big fan of continuing to take the pill and missing a period that way, for months, which some girls do. But I'd start manipulating them using the pill and so my two key dates were always Gotzis [the world heptathlon competition] and the Championships and I'd work backwards from there to find out when my periods would be and then change them.'

What Marilyn and Kelly discovered, through trial and error, is that periods cause most havoc to an athlete's body in the week leading up to bleeding. Dr Charlotte Cowie, Clinical Director at St George's Park, has worked with every kind of athlete from Olympians to Premier League footballers and has seen the impact periods can have on sportswomen. But she tells me that she feels hesitant to speak about it because for most women the benefits of exercising before and during a period far outweigh any negative side effects. 'I do agree it's a real step forward being able to talk about this stuff, but we've got to put it into context: statistically women who don't exercise regularly are much more likely to have symptoms of menstrual pain than women who do exercise regularly and my worry would be that a big discussion around [the negative effects] would make women think it's not OK or it's difficult to train when they're menstruating. When actually it's just so important for women to exercise. There are some studies in relation to injury rates and women who are menstruating, though . . . it seems there are points in the menstrual cycle where you are more prone to injury.'

Charlotte says some of the more common problems she sees are practical ones, things that might affect any woman – not just athletes. She talks about training facilities where the toilets cater for men only and yet women have to change their sanitary protection there. For young girls, only just coming into puberty, this can create an extra barrier to them doing sport and exercise. 'For young athletes, just remembering to have the appropriate sanitary protection is important so they're not worrying about it and are prepared so they don't have that fear they'll suddenly be caught competing and there's nothing they can do about it.' For elite athletes of any age, the drugs tester visits feel particularly intrusive when they are on their period. Drugs testers are expected to 'watch where the wee comes from', as Kelly puts it, to ensure that urine samples are genuine. But for a woman on her period this can feel humiliating. There might be blood in the urine, or a visible tampon thread, or a full sanitary pad in your underwear. Thank goodness, then, that the testers are at least female. Tanni Grey-Thompson remembers a time in her career, in the 1980s and 1990s, when she occasionally had to provide samples in front of male doctors.

Treating the common symptoms of menstruation, such as period pain, can usually be achieved with normal painkillers. But while many women prefer to use alternative remedies such as evening primrose oil, these can be problematic for elite athletes who need every medication they take to be batch tested in order to prevent doping test complications. 'In terms of hormonal manipulation it's an individual thing, if girls are very young and they're not sexually active yet it's a big step for them to start taking the pill. Whereas if someone's in a relationship and they need a method of contraception anyway then they can more appropriately consider going on the pill,' says Charlotte.

Each sport has its own challenges – Olympic athletes have just one tiny window every four years to perform, compared to footballers who compete the year round, or tennis players who need to peak at least four times a year for the Grand Slams. 'If you're in a weight-regulated sport like weightlifting or tae kwon do you don't want to be dealing with water retention ahead of a major competition,' says Charlotte, 'so there's individual solutions for individual athletes. There's only a tiny percentage of athletes who have terrible symptoms. That's why I feel so sorry for Heather Watson, because not only is it very hard to talk about, but because it's not that common she may not have had other female tennis players to talk to about it. Having looked after the whole England women's football squad, there were a few players who took anti-inflammatories but only one athlete who really struggled with severe performance-limiting pain. So it's not nothing, but it's certainly not the majority.' Indeed, Charlotte, who previously worked at the Lawn Tennis Association, believes that tennis players have it hardest, being on the road for most of the year, searching for sanitary protection in different countries around the world, and not having the same doctor throughout the season, as medics are assigned to specific tournaments rather than to athletes. It's an opinion shared by Judy Murray, former captain of the British Fed Cup team which includes Heather. 'Because the women's tour is so dominated by men, especially if your coach is a single guy, the whole thing with periods becomes a very difficult thing to explain because it's not something a man will ever experience himself,' Judy tells me. 'So if they're not close to someone who has to deal with that every month – a wife, girlfriend, partner – many of them won't get it. But it's a fact of life that significantly affects performance at certain times of a player's cycle so we need to make sure they do understand the ins and outs of that and we shouldn't be afraid of talking about it.'

Then, quite unexpectedly, Charlotte reveals something that stops me in my tracks. Research around periods and injuries, she says, has only been taking place in the last decade. I am so stunned I ask her to repeat this fact. 'Yes, well, most of the studies that we go on in sport are nearly always on male subjects and so we make assumptions about female athletes in relation to research being done on males.' But how can this be? How can male bodies be so casually substituted for female bodies? Charlotte matter-of-factly explains that there are fewer elite sportswomen than sportsmen, and fewer women exercising than men, which makes recruitment for research trials more challenging. And then there's the money factor. 'Generally speaking male sports are better funded so there's more financial support to do research on male athletes than female athletes.' But there must be so much we don't know about the female body then, I ask? 'Very much so, yes,' says Charlotte.

This is a bombshell. Men's bodies being substituted for female bodies in sports research is about as unscientific as you can get. A few weeks later I go to see the campaigner and journalist Caroline Criado-Perez, best known for protesting against the Bank of England's decision to remove Elizabeth Fry from the £5 note, leaving no female presence on English banknotes. Caroline's protest captured the public's imagination because what was a relatively small detail in our currency snowballed into a national campaign. Soon politicians were up in arms and both Caroline and the MP Stella Creasy received rape and death threats for their audacity in speaking out.

When we meet, Caroline tells me she is writing a column about this exact issue in science. 'It's the kind of sexism I find most interesting, when the male is the default,' she explains. She tells me about crash test dummies that were based on male bodies for decades, until someone realized they'd better find out the impact on pregnant women's bodies. 'It's the same thing with drugs; the FDA [the US Food and Drug Administration] have had to cut the dosage of sleeping pills for women in half because women's bodies metabolize the active ingredients much quicker. They only just realized this in 2013.' But Caroline hasn't finished yet. 'And then there's the women who were being misdiagnosed when they presented with heart attacks because they had different symptoms from men and lots of doctors had been only trained in male symptoms, so they'd send them off home thinking they had stomach or indigestion problems. Of course no doctor wants to misdiagnose a woman, but it's happening because of the way the female body is seen as the male body with some boobs tacked on. Female medicine is just about female troubles, rather than seeing our whole body as different.

'The most astonishing thing was the rationale behind not testing on women which was that the female body is too hormonal. That's very interesting to me on a number of bases. If a test cannot account for the bodies of 50 per cent of the population, surely there's something wrong with the test, not the bodies. But the male body also fluctuates hormonally, so the science is incorrect. So it doesn't make sense in any way. I find it so fascinating that even scientists who are interested in fact are basing their decisions on incorrect methods.'

We sit there in silence for a moment digesting this thought: how can science be so unscientific? In the weeks that follow I come across dozens more examples. There's the alcohol test for the controversial female Viagra pill, which used twenty-three men and just two women for one of its trials despite the fact that women have a lower tolerance of alcohol than men. And the article I read in US publication the *Atlantic* about a woman who went to the ER in severe pain and waited nine hours to get a diagnosis while medical staff told her to calm down, stop crying and wait her turn. It turned out she had ovarian torsion and was hours away from death. The article says that women's symptoms are routinely played down in the US medical system compared to those of male patients. In the US, 'men wait an average of 49 minutes before receiving an analgesic for acute abdominal pain. Women wait an average of 65 minutes for the same thing.'[18]

What is clear is that women need answers, they need guidance. They need the science, and they need it right now. Marilyn is thirty-one at the time I am writing this book. This is probably the last major championship cycle of her career. She's already missed out on so much expertise. It's so unjust. 'It's not that female athletes are looking for an excuse,' she says, 'but not having awareness of your movement [in your menstrual cycle] is dangerous. It's simple things like wearing compression leggings or a sacroiliac belt to keep my hip movement in check. If there are things out there that can help me I want to have the knowledge and not just find out using trial and error, which it's been like – I mean it's literally been me on the Internet googling stuff.' I can't help but think this is mad. Can you picture Wayne Rooney or Usain Bolt sitting at their laptops desperately googling solutions to their medical problems? It just wouldn't happen.

I need to speak to an expert. As it happens a consultant gynaecologist for the International Olympic Committee is giving a speech to the British Association of Sport and Exercise Medicine, titled 'To Bleed or not to Bleed? That is the Question!' Mr Michael Dooley appears to be the leading expert in this country on sport and menstruation.

Over the next four months I speak to Michael every few weeks. I have never met anyone so passionate, or who speaks with such fervour, about the health of the female body. He's worked with some of Britain's most famous sportswomen – from Paula Radcliffe to Mary King – both of whom have written about the support he has given them through their pregnancies. He wants to tell the world about periods, infertility, pregnancy, the menopause, the benefits of exercise and the health of a woman. Despite spending years devoting his professional career to this subject, I quickly discover over the course of our conversations that there remain a lot of unanswered questions in this area. 'Sadly there are no answers to a lot of your questions because we don't have all the evidence,' he says. 'That's what I'm trying to do, more research. I'm probably one of the only gynaecologists in England looking at elite and recreational athletes because it is such an important area to be addressed.'

But *why* isn't there more research, I ask, exasperated. 'Because we're quite a conservative lot, the medical community, only recently are we realizing the importance of exercise and sport,' he says. 'In my lifetime we've had a huge cultural shift around attitudes to women and exercise – from only 11 per cent of the athletes competing at the 1960 Olympics being female, to 42 per cent at London 2012. Therefore we have moved very quickly socially, but we haven't taken it on medically, and we're only beginning to realize the benefits of being active. Even culturally, though, I still don't think that we're encouraging women to compete or take part in exercise at any level.' Michael says a lack of investment in research is a big part of the problem, and he is working towards setting up the first ever NHS sports gynaecology clinic to extend his work in the private sector.

'There's no doubt that premenstrual syndrome can be greatly improved by doing exercise, ditto endometriosis and pelvic pain

– and we're not talking about the elite here, everyone can bene-fit – and there's no doubt fertility can be improved by losing weight because too much body fat affects your hormones. So an educational programme isn't too difficult but we also need more data on what the problems are – I've got quite a huge database now from athletes coming to me with their problems. Five years ago I was saying to people with low body fat that being on the pill is fine. Now there is evidence that this may not be the case and that the combined oral contraceptive may not be as benefi-cial for bone protection as we thought. The newer contraceptive pills, which contain natural oestrogen, may be better.'

Michael's specialist area is elite athletes, but his message that this issue affects all women – not just sporty ones – is important. At school, and as a young woman, I remember the terrible pain that many of my friends went through prior to and during menstruation. They were in and out of the doctor's surgery, being put on different drugs to control the symptoms. I was lucky never to suffer in that way; it looked excruciating. During that time they were never given advice to exercise – right at the point in their lives when they most needed to engage with physical activity, and when they were most at risk of being lost to sport and exercise forever. Instead all the talk was of hot-water bottles and curling up in bed, enduring the cramps. Imagine if they had been told that exercise would alleviate their pain? Why don't we convey these messages in schools? Why don't we educate young women – whether they're walking into a GP's surgery, or reading a magazine?

Out of the blue, Michael asks me if I've read *The Diary of Anne Frank*. Yes, I say, confused as to what the Nazi occupation has to do with periods. 'Well,' he says, 'that's well worth reading because she talks a lot about periods. She says: *I don't like them but they're my inner secret* – and that's very important because that's so true. When someone comes along and tells me "I've got regular periods," instantly I know what's going on with someone's hormones.' The point that Michael is making is that women – all women – need to be able to talk about their periods because they tell us so much. Rather than shying away from them as some sort of taboo, we should be positively embracing them, grateful for everything they can tell us about our own bodies. 'We've got to educate women about their own reproductive health. The number of talks I give to women, highly intelligent, high-powered women, who don't understand their own body, they didn't understand that after menopause they didn't need contraception, they didn't understand the risks of the menopause. Women don't know what happens during ovulation, or during PMS, there's a huge lack of understanding, even very basic things which if they did understand could really help to prevent lots of problems.'

What about sex, I say? How does sex impact on a woman's athletic performance? Is it like what they say about men? That sex and orgasms weaken the testosterone and therefore abstinence is the best approach for athletes? Michael says he doesn't know. He hasn't come across any research about women, sport and sex.

It's not just Michael. Everyone I ask, from medics to athletes, tells me the same thing. And, crucially, most say they've never thought about it before. And so I find myself stumbling into the next information black hole.

Some years ago I was asked to write an article about sex and sport for *Observer Sport Monthly*. There was the usual hype at the time around the Beijing 2008 Olympic Games and how many crates of condoms would be made available to horny athletes whose libido had been boosted by intense athletic competition. Was it all an irresistible urban myth? Or was there any truth in it? A British sprinter, who requested to remain anonymous, spilled the beans and described corridors full of girls queuing for a night of passion with male athletes after competition. But, interestingly, he also talked about his female teammates. 'Some of the girls say they can't compete unless they've had sex the night before an event. One girl told me she feels lighter on her feet after sex and has a greater sense of well-being.'[19]

I need to ask a female athlete if this is folklore, or whether there's any truth at all in it. But how many sportswomen are going to talk to a journalist about their sex lives? Hmm. If there's one woman you can ask anything it's Kelly Sotherton, Olympic bronze-medal-winning heptathlete and famous for having bold opinions. I relay the anonymous sprinter's story to Kelly and she laughs her head off. 'Those sprinters are lying!' she roars. 'Honestly! I think the media has made the Olympics out to be an orgy. People get a little bit drunk and some people might have sex, of course they do, but not everyone goes to the Olympics, gets ten condoms and uses them!'

However Kelly does admit that sex talk is more common among athletes than we might think. She says one of her coaches used to give practical advice to the group on ensuring that sex did not get in the way of athletic performance. 'We do have these open conversations, we talk about it down the track. If you were a fly on the wall you'd write about twenty books,' she cackles. 'It's stuff like if the guy's standing up then he's using his legs more so he'll be fatigued; you wouldn't want to do that ahead of a competition, so my coach would just say which positions to avoid and that sort of thing. But I think it all depends on the person, their make-up, physiology and mindset.'

Kelly suggests that many male athletes are less sexually active between April and September, during the outdoor competitive season, though she admits that much of this is down to superstition, rather than scientific fact. 'If you are in the shape of your life and you've trained hard the only thing that's going to be detrimental to your performance is if you've had no sleep. But if you're home with your partner and you've done it and it's not very long, you're probably OK,' she laughs. Which chimes with some of the advice doled out to national teams ahead of the recent men's World Cup in Brazil, where French players were permitted to have sex only if they didn't stay up all night, or the Nigerian team who were allegedly told only to have sex with their wives (because, some say, it's the looking for sex and lack of sleep that's the problematic part, not the act itself).

I want to know: does the same apply to female athletes? 'I don't really know,' says Kelly. 'I think some female athletes probably would abstain a little bit before a competition. Saying that, if you told them they would throw 10m further in the javelin or one tenth of a second faster over 100m if they had sex the night before, I'm sure they would all be doing it to win a few more medals!' One athlete who believes it definitely has an impact is Ultimate Fighting Championship (UFC) star Ronda Rousey. 'For girls, it raises your testosterone,' she says, 'so I try to have as much sex as possible before I fight actually. Not with everybody. I don't put out like a Craigslist ad or anything, but if I got a steady, I'm going to be like, "Yo, fight time's coming up."'[20]

I ask Kelly, and others, if it works the other way around – if women exercise more, does it actually *increase* their libido? The consensus seems to be that, psychologically, working out helps women to feel more confident about their bodies, and that in turn makes them more inclined to want to have sex. It's all about being connected to your physicality, and feeling positive about that connection.

But what if there's something more? I mean, what *physical* effect does exercise have on a woman's body when it comes to sex, and vice versa? Scouring the Internet for solutions brought up scant evidence, until Michael mentioned in passing something he had read in *The Times*. Suzi Godson, the newspaper's resident Q&A expert, answered a letter from a forty-five-year-old woman who had recently got into fitness and running marathons and discovered an increased libido. The only problem was her husband couldn't keep up with her. Suzi cited a number of studies that show exercise for men increases their levels of testosterone and stamina in the bedroom – from as young as eighteen right through to middle age. So far, so familiar. But what interested me most about Suzi's answer was her reference to the changes for women when they exercised. 'A lot of fascinating studies have shown that exercise has significant sexual benefits for women,' she wrote. 'One study showed that female athletes have better sexual function and more efficient clitoral blood flow than healthy sedentary females — but you don't need to be an Olympian to experience the sexual rewards of exercise.'[21]

This last point is really important. If exercise can boost a woman's sex drive then we may have stumbled on a significant breakthrough for women who are currently struggling with libido, whether through medical or hormonal conditions such as the menopause, psychosexual problems, or just being stressed out and not having the time or the energy. At a time when the world is racing towards a chemical solution in the form of the controversial pill – female Viagra – perhaps there is an easier, healthier, safer option right under our noses? After all, isn't sex just about connecting mind to body? But in western society, where we are led by our brains all day – from work to social media and technology – we are surely in need of more 'body time'? I know when I exercise after a period of being sedentary, I feel like my body is waking up. I suddenly remember all these parts of myself – my feet! My neck! My spine! We use our bodies all day long, of course, but we do it in a very disconnected way. I can't help feeling that someone should be researching this.

In recent years there has, at least, been more interest in trying to solve the 'mystery' of the female orgasm. Some of these studies have made incidental discoveries that relate to female athletes and physically active women. In a famous case, the American distance runner Lynn Jennings broke an age-old taboo after winning the US 10km title in 1993. Lynn reportedly attributed her victory to having had sex the night before, saying it 'solidifies my core feeling of happiness'. A few years later the Israeli scientist Alexander Olshanietzky confirmed this notion, hitting the headlines with his conclusion that female athletes performed better at sporting events when they had orgasmed the night before. 'We believe that a woman gets better results in sports competition after orgasm,' he said at the time. 'Generally, it's true of high jumpers and runners. The more orgasms, the more chances of winning a medal. Coaches generally tell their athletes to abstain before competition. In the case of women, that's the wrong advice.'[22]

Meanwhile, in 2006, psychology professor Barry Komisaruk and sex therapist Beverley Whittle teamed up for a ground-breaking scientific experiment at Rutgers University to measure how pain thresholds were altered by vaginal self-stimulation in women. Incredibly, they found that masturbation doubled the pain threshold of women. In a subsequent study the academics went on to look at pain thresholds during childbirth and found a correlation between the baby emerging through the birth canal, around the area of the G-spot, better enabling the birth process and ultimately helping mothers to bond with their newborn babies. Spurred on, they began to study women with spinal cord injuries who had been told by doctors they would never again experience sensation from vaginal or clitoral stimulation. Whittle and Komisaruk proved this theory wrong, mapping out the pathways between female genitalia and the brain.

What does all of this mean for athletes, or for women who exercise? It's still pretty unclear, unfortunately. But the concept of orgasm or vaginal stimulation reducing physical pain in women is an interesting one and, if further explored, could completely change the way we talk about sex and exercise to women of all levels of physical activity. Already some running magazines and exercise publications are interpreting the research as significant to women's physical activity – speculating that those painful long runs could be relieved by an orgasm or two. Whether that's a true interpretation of the research or not, the developments underline why science must pursue greater knowledge of women's bodies across the board as opposed to relying on male bodies for a default conclusion on the human race. And if exercise and sport can really boost a woman's libido then what a brilliant, health-inducing method to adopt. Give me an aerobics class over a pill any day! Focusing on these avenues could provide the kind of research that might prove life-changing for women everywhere.

Whenever we talk about sport and exercise for women, we habitually talk about girls, or young women in their twenties and thirties. But what about everyone else? Have we already given up on women over forty? Over fifty? What about women like my mum, now in her seventies? One of the most moving moments in my research was meeting Sport England CEO Jennie Price. I have to be honest and say that the idea of interviewing a CEO doesn't usually fill me with much interest. But as Jennie sits down, *Star Wars* notebook in hand, there is something different about her; she has a life story to tell.

Jennie grew up with a professional sportsman for a dad (a footballer for Wolverhampton Wanderers) but she never really played any organized team sport. In fact, she wasn't very physically active at all until one day, in her thirties, when she was experiencing a lot of stress in her job and a male friend suggested she start going to the gym. This scenario rings true for many women, who so often only find exercise later in their lives. Ten happy years followed working out at the gym (a place she had previously been terrified of, until the young man doing the induction told her to ignore all the intimidating-looking people in Lycra: 'They're only really looking at themselves.') But on relocating to a new area, Jennie suddenly found that her exercise routine went out of the window. She couldn't find another gym that she liked, or the facilities weren't convenient to her new life. Hers is a familiar tale to many women who so easily fall off

– and then struggle to get back on – the exercise wagon. Eventually, though, Jennie discovered power walking and soon fell in love with exercising all over again.

Until, one day, something horrible happened that threatened to shatter her confidence completely, and almost stopped her from exercising in public altogether. 'After all those years in the gym I got very used to wrapping a cloak around me thinking no one's looking at me,' says Jennie. 'So I wasn't expecting anybody to take any notice anytime I went out. On this particular occasion, for some stupid reason, I'd left my phone at home and I happened to be the furthest distance from home in my walk. And as I powered along this man came to the front of his shop – a fast-food joint – opened the door and shouted at me. Well, I won't say what he shouted, but it had a lot of swear words. He waved and gestured and shouted. And I suddenly realized, "Oh my God, he's shouting at me! Maybe I look terrible. Maybe I shouldn't be out here, maybe everyone is thinking, my God, what's she doing?" And it was horrible. I walked home and burst into tears when I got in.' Jennie was so embarrassed she didn't tell her husband for two weeks. 'Isn't that awful?' she says. 'I felt ashamed.' Why ashamed? 'Because I thought maybe I do look awful, maybe I shouldn't be exercising in public. Maybe I do look ridiculous – I must look ridiculous if somebody did that. I thought maybe I won't do it any more. Then I thought, for God's sake, Jennie, you're raising thousands of pounds for breast cancer, get over yourself. So I went back out, but I was nervous.'

Jennie's experience took place before the launch of Sport England's groundbreaking This Girl Can campaign, encouraging women and girls to be physically active. But it was during the research and creative process for the campaign that the message being put out there suddenly hit home. This wasn't just a campaign, this was relevant to Jennie's own personal life. 'When we did the judgement research [a Sport England survey found that 75 per cent of women wanted to take part in sport but were worried about being judged] and they brought the picture of the man staring at the woman running . . .' Jennie takes a sharp breath, 'well, I thought, oh yes, I recognize that.'

At the official launch of the campaign, Jennie decided to tell her story to a packed roomful of people. 'I didn't intend to,' she says now. 'I had a script and that story wasn't in it. But I looked at that audience and I suddenly thought: I know what this feels like and I probably need to admit that. I want them to connect to this emotionally so I'm going to take the risk. I think it kind of sealed people's connection and made them realize I was doing this for the right reasons, not just because it's my job. And This Girl Can is the thing I've done professionally that I feel most emotionally connected to. If you didn't pay me I'd still want to work on this campaign because I really recognize this stuff. I've been that chubby girl, I've been the woman at the treadmill standing there thinking, "Oh my God." I've been through all of that stuff and I've always felt very inadequate because of it. And that stuff really matters to me.'

As I listen to Jennie's story I think about the fact that she's a woman in her fifties. I hadn't really considered what it is like to be in your fifties and facing these challenges. Even This Girl Can's target audience doesn't extend beyond women in their early forties. And then, quite unexpectedly, we find ourselves talking about a taboo that, as a woman in my thirties, I hadn't planned on writing about at all. That taboo is the menopause.

It's Jennie who is first to bring it up. 'I don't talk about this normally,' she says carefully, 'but it is quite scary, particularly when you edge towards things like the menopause, because your body changes as much as it changes in adolescence but people don't talk about it very much, and so you shove it aside in your daily life. You know, I sit in meetings and have hot flushes and we all pretend it's not happening,' she laughs. I laugh. But I don't really know what she is talking about. Yes, I've heard of hot flushes – but not *really*. Not really like I know anything much about them.

'Put that in an exercise context, and you're not quite as resilient as you were, it's not as easy to control your weight, there's stuff going on in your body that you're worried about, and you do have another raft of things to cope with. It's really tempting to think, oh, [exercise] is not relevant to me any more, all the stuff about the excitement and the fun side of exercise, that's not for me any more, I think that's a really strongly held view. And if I sit through another sports seminar where people say, "Oh, I think we should give bowling to the over-fifties" . . . I'm fifty-five, for God's sake, I do not want to bowl just yet! I can still do plenty of other things! And I think we need more women standing up and saying that kind of stuff.'

We do. I tell Jennie that I hope the next phase of the campaign embraces older women (the current campaign is aimed at fourteen- to forty-year-olds). Later I contact a precursor of This Girl Can, a pilot project called 'I Will If You Will', an experiment in how to get an entire town of women and girls physically active, based in Bury. I hear about the case studies, such as seventy-one-year-old Anne who's taken up boxing and loves it, and about Boogie Bounce, where the instructors are open about what happens to postnatal women, or women of a certain age, who jump about on trampolines. They have a giggle about it. A we're-all-in-this-together type camaraderie. They remind women to go to the toilet before the class starts, or make sure their Tena Lady pads are in.

I'm so grateful to have been put on the right track by Jennie, to be thinking about women over forty. If the average life expectancy of a woman in the UK is eighty-one years, then why on earth are we ignoring half of our lifespan? Is age really that much of a taboo? And if we're failing girls and women in their twenties and thirties when it comes to getting them physically active, then surely we need to capture the women who got away – those in their forties, fifties, sixties and beyond, who might yet adopt the kind of lifestyle that would bring them happiness and greater health.

For a lot of women, like Jennie Price, the reality is that women often find exercise later in life. And sometimes, that's precisely when they need it most. I recently read the life story of Emma Bridgewater, the British ceramicist mogul whose crockery adorns pretty much every dresser in middle England. Now in her fifties, Emma eulogizes over the importance of exercise for women – often juggling a career and a family – who desperately need an outlet for such full and demanding lives. 'If you don't look after yourself, very simply, and definitely, you will get ill,' she wrote in her autobiography. 'I hammered on without heeding the distress signals until my immune system suffered, after which I developed a mild form of rheumatoid arthritis, which I still ignored and soon I found I was pretty much immobilized.' Emma now exercises every day, and has become evangelical about the benefits. 'Roughly speaking you need to feel normal again by the end of every day, and don't let the pressure build up. A swim, a run or, really best of all, a walk, is a good way to shake off the stress which accumulates during the day.'[23]

I phone Michael – what does he know about the menopause and exercise? 'I've written a book about it!' he practically yells down the phone. 'Exercise is good for age. For men and women. But for women the added risk of the menopause is osteoporosis, there are dreadful stats – it's a killer.' I frown. A killer? My grandmother had it, and began to hunch over in her eighties. It was horrible to see, but I didn't think it had killed her. Isn't osteoporosis the deterioration of the bones? 'Yes, but it's a silent killer because once you have had an osteoporotic fracture there is a significant increased risk of death rate. This can be associ-ated with complications following the fracture and increased immobility.' Michael says weight-bearing exercise is best for supporting bone density – running, tennis, the gym, but not swimming (although that's good aerobic exercise), while any-thing cardiovascular will help with preventing cardiovascular problems, such as weight gain and type 2 diabetes. 'Exercise isn't enough to prevent osteoporosis on its own. But because you're fitter with stronger muscles you're less likely to fall, and there-fore less likely to suffer an osteoporotic fracture. I once asked a patient if she did much exercise and she looked at me and said, "I don't do movement, Michael." She's eighty-nine now and bright as a button, but totally immobilized due to loss of height and severe spinal curvature. It's dreadful.'

Michael sings the praises of exercise for combating some of the symptoms of the menopause, particularly depression. And when I ask him about hot flushes he recommends a yoga exer-cise. 'Hot flushes are often stimulated by a stressful situation; there's a thing called alternate nose breathing. People who are about to give a talk or at committee meetings, if they sit and breathe through alternate nostrils, in through the left and out through the right, that decreases your stress and cortisol and your hot flushes.'

Later that evening my mum calls and I tell her about my conversations. 'Mum, the menopause sounds so scary,' I say. 'Oh, Anna,' she says, 'you don't need to worry about any of that. You're pregnant! And you've got years before the menopause starts.' But I make a quick calculation in my head, and I haven't got years. Not really. I'm thirty-seven. If the menopause starts in my early fifties, say, then that's only as far away as my mid twenties, which, quite frankly, feels like only the other day. How can this huge, life-changing event be hovering just a few years ahead of me, and I know absolutely nothing about it? Why is nobody talking about this stuff? My mum tells me a bit of what she knows – she talks about HRT (Hormone Replacement Therapy) and depression and weight gain and osteoporosis. Then there's incontinence and vaginal dryness. I say, 'Mum, it feels like when you're a kid and you find out about periods, or when you're a young woman and you go through childbirth and realize that the whole world has been keeping this monumental secret from you.' 'Yes,' says my mum, 'it is a bit like that.' I go to bed thinking about the menopause and what it might mean for me. Suddenly life seems very different.

5

How to avoid the pregnant pause

When Jessica Ennis-Hill announced her pregnancy in January 2014, the chorus of opinion accompanying the news was all too familiar. 'Will she still have the ambition for it?' ran the bulletins. 'Is this the end of her career?' It was like hearing a million of our own bosses, amplified across national TV and radio.

That's part of what made watching Jess's world championship victory in Beijing so glorious – not only did she beat the world's best heptathletes on the track, she beat the world's biggest doubters off it. Her victory was our victory, and an enormous leap towards reassessing the way we routinely portray mums as washed-up human beings who can just about string a sentence together and struggle to brush their hair. Not that we need to have fabulous hair all the time. Nice hair is not helping with the need for more female presidents, neuroscientists and businesswomen. Nice hair is not going to bridge the pay gap, ladies!

Watching Jess's gold-medal-winning performance, just thirteen months after she gave birth to her son Reggie, was emotional. My eyes pricked with tears; I had a lump in my throat. Women's sport does that to me anyway. But Jess's world title meant more. It was such a calm, confident, perfectly formed riposte to anyone who had thought she was a write-off. What a woman. 'Woman?' said my husband. 'She's a superhuman!' And it was special to see the look of awe on his face. But super-human? Paradoxically, in my eyes at least, becoming a mother had made Jess more human than ever. Motherhood had brought her – and her incredible six-pack – that little bit closer to all of us. Because here was a person who had just been through a year of disorientating sleep patterns, maternity pads, leaky boobs, mopping sick off your clothes, trying to stick to a routine, jug-gling childcare and work, and ultimately feeling torn between wanting to devote your entire life to this tiny human being, and wanting to remain a person in your own right who can still achieve remarkable things. And she still went out, and rocked it.

Over the years I have marvelled at the powerful transition Jess has undergone, from the twenty-one-year-old I first met in a sandwich shop in Sheffield many years ago, to the almighty cultural icon she is today. Back then I was interviewing Jessica Ennis, as she used to be known, as an up-and-coming track and field star. There were no PR people present, just Jess, sitting on a stool munching on a panini. She talked about her construction-worker boyfriend (now husband) Andy, her university degree in psychology, shopping with friends. She was smiley and lovely, chatty and down to earth.

Since then she has developed into the most incredible, near indomitable, athlete. As an athletics correspondent, between 2008 and 2012, I relished seeing her compete: whether that was a windy spring afternoon in front of fifty people in Cudworth,

South Yorkshire, or on a glorious track in front of thousands in New York. What I admired most was her champion's ability to change a performance, bounce back from disappointments, excel in her weakest events just when she most needed to pull something out of the bag. Not many athletes can do that. And she always went about it so quietly, with a modest little skip and a smile to celebrate each new success across the seven events. Soon Jess and her perfectly formed abdominals became world famous. But she never really changed. She'd sit down for an interview and offer you some hand cream ('It's such a good one,' she'd say, pulling a tube of Elizabeth Arden out of her kitbag and squirting out a generous blob), or she'd ask about your partner, your pregnancy, your new handbag. She could relate to anybody and everybody, the people's princess of sport. And then she'd discreetly zoom off – in a sports car fit for a sports star, a trail of schoolboys running after her shouting, 'We love you, Jess!' and you'd suddenly remember just what a stellar act she was.

The fact that Jess was brave enough to become a mother at the height of her career speaks volumes. And I do mean brave. I remember one top female athlete describing how coaches often pressured sportswomen into delaying starting a family, because children were seen as an inconvenience to their careers. It's the same in the workplace, of course. I'd previously been told, with a grin, 'Don't get pregnant!' Or there was the former boss who went on a rant about, 'everyone having fucking children in this office!' which he seemed particularly keen to share with me.

And that's why Jess should be an icon for all working mums. Because women who have children are still seen as a drain on the resources of a workplace. It should be a national scandal that in the UK 54,000 women a year lose their jobs due to maternity discrimination, and yet too many people still think women are deceiving their employers by getting pregnant, conning them into handouts. They still think that women who get pregnant are letting everyone down, and that once they return to work they will have transformed into useless, baby-obsessed, empty-headed zombies. Even if you're not a mother, cannot have children, or don't intend ever to have children, the repercussions of this trend are felt by all women.

After having my daughter I was shocked at the sheer number of horror stories I heard at playgroups from lawyers, teachers, architects, journalists, marketing execs, in one case even a woman employed at a leading equality organization. And yet where is the government rhetoric? Where are the campaigns? There's an awful lot of talk about affordable childcare, but no one seems to question the bigger picture: why don't we actually *value* mothers in the workplace? This *Lean In* business is all very well, but mothers can't 'lean' unless they're supported. As the 'first lady of football' Karren Brady once told me, 'I love employing mums, they're extremely organized and efficient. They have to be.' So why do we keep making it so hard for them?

For now, in Britain at least, it seems to be sportswomen who are leading the way for mothers as empowering figures. We've had the air-punching inspirational story of Jo Pavey, who at forty and with two young children became a household name when she won the first ever major gold medal of her career. I had to laugh, reading about her handwashing the kids' clothes and drying them on a windowsill during the European Championships in Zurich. And how can you not beam when she repeatedly says it was having her kids that gave her the happiness to finally excel on a major stage? I wanted to leap up and hug Jo every time she said that, because it's a message we need to be getting out there loud and clear: having kids is not the end of your life. Women can achieve wonderful things as mothers. And it's nothing to do with that ridiculous guilt-inducing expression, 'having it all'; it's just about being proud of who we are as mums and having the confidence and support to go on to achieve amazing things, rather than being cast as muddled snivelling wrecks.

I know some people find the whole motherhood and sportswomen stories thing patronizing. They argue: why can't we just hear about their sporting achievements? Why do we need to know that they breastfed, or that they battled with pre-eclampsia? Women give birth every day, it's no big deal. Well, I actually think it is a huge deal. It is such a huge deal that every father or partner I've ever met is overcome with awe and newfound respect for all women after having watched their other half go through the process. Because birth, in all of its forms, is a physical trauma. And, no, birth and motherhood shouldn't be how we define sportswomen in that myopic way, but celebrating these stories publicly is a good thing. Because, for the most part, the physical reality of birth – and recovering from it – is hidden away. In films and TV series we only ever see a bit of huffing and puffing, maybe some screaming, and then there's a cute baby and it's all over.

But that's not the end of it. Birth is just the beginning, and I don't mean all the challenges around adjusting to a new baby, but the physical trauma that affects postnatal women, whether they've had a vaginal birth and are struggling with stitches and incontinence, or have to cope with a caesarean scar that prevents them from lifting or even driving for at least six weeks after the birth. Then there's diastasis recti which is when your abdominals don't grow back together properly after pregnancy – a condition that is thought to affect one-third of women and causes chronic back pain – cracked and bleeding nipples, migraines from epidurals and recovering from episiotomy. As one local exercise teacher, who specializes in mothers returning to exercise post-birth, told me, 'having a baby is like recovering from an injury'.

All of which makes life after birth a huge hurdle for mums. And it doesn't help that we don't get to hear enough about the very physical reality of those experiences and how they impact on a woman's body. That's why I was so pleased to write up the story of former England rugby hooker and mother of one, Emma Croker, and her return to an international rugby career.[24] Emma had a caesarean and was advised to wait four months before going back to training because of the additional recovery time required. As she counted the days until her return, Emma admits she was terrified of how her internal wounds would hold up to the physicality of rugby. So she did the only thing she could think of to dispel her fears. She ordered her teammate Becky Essex to run at her midriff with all her strength. Bam! Somehow the wound survived. 'My pain threshold increased after having a baby,' laughed Emma afterwards. Despite the fact that over 25 per cent of women in the UK give birth by caesarean – and a whopping 50 per cent in Brazil – it's a subject for which the realities are rarely discussed in public. Indeed, I'm pretty sure that's the first time any national newspaper has published a major article in a sports section about a C-section. I can still remember the phone call with my editor after I filed the copy. There was a pause, and a sniff. 'There's, um, a lot about caesareans in there,' he said quietly. 'Yes!' I enthused. 'And isn't it such an amazing story?' To his credit, he didn't change a word.

Of course, stories about motherhood are not always uplifting, because motherhood isn't always uplifting. Sometimes it's one almighty struggle. And if we don't tell those stories we can't bring about change. Take the example of Katie Chapman, England's star midfielder for over a decade, who says she was effectively forced to retire from international duty ahead of the 2011 World Cup because she couldn't afford the childcare. The equivalent would have been Steven Gerrard saying he had to give up his England career because he needed to look after the kids. That, of course, would never have happened because Stevie G. is paid enough money to cover the childcare costs of every woman in the England team. Female footballers, however, often have to work alongside their playing career just to make ends meet. Wages have gone up substantially in women's football since then, but I still find it embarrassing that the FA shrugged their shoulders as one of their star players was forced to sit out the biggest tournament in the world because of childcare costs.

By way of comparison, in the United States the women's national team has an entirely different approach. The head coach, World Cup-winning Jill Ellis, is a mother, as are some of the star names in the team – from Christie Rampone to Shannon Boxx. The federation pays childcare expenses, from nannies to travel and accommodation. And the kids come with the team. There are kids in the hotel, kids in the dressing room and kids in the canteen. Obviously there are boundaries; they are not running free, and World Cup and Olympic finals are exempt from the arrangements, but if mothers haven't had to pay expenses for all the training camps, friendlies and other tournaments the year round it's not going to be so hard to pay for the championships that occur only once every four years.

The English FA have improved their maternity offerings since 2011 and Katie was able to return to the international fold for the 2015 World Cup in Canada. But the lack of financial – and cultural – support still makes it hard for mums. Neither defender Casey Stoney, mother of twins; or Katie, who has three young sons, could afford to bring their children out to Canada for the tournament. Had there been more support the rest of the year perhaps they might have been able to.

Inevitably some will ask: why should an employer pay for kids to be around? It's not their responsibility. No, but then listen to what Jill Ellis told me: 'I think it's great, it shows how much respect the female athletes have over here. Sometimes my daughter will come on trips; I love it, it keeps the dynamic light. It's actually a bonus to have kids around – the players are professional and they understand the parameters. It's awesome: you've got a high chair over here, you've got one running around over there. In the locker room the kids are dancing – you see the players light up.'[25] If that approach can help win you a World Cup . . .

OK, so most of us wouldn't think of bringing our babies to work, but then again, why not? Journalist Afua Hirsch wrote a fascinating report for the *Guardian* some years back about mothers working in Ghana. 'The reality is that most women here have a very simple solution to the challenge of working motherhood. They just strap their babies on to their backs and carry on.'[26] At the time Afua had a one-year-old baby and was

Ghana correspondent, a role that most of her colleagues thought incompatible with motherhood. But her reflections on the cultural differences were profound. 'I've noticed that African women don't waste much time feeling guilty about the inevitable imperfect situations that come with being a working mother,' she wrote, and my God, is that a sentence that will stop many western mothers in their tracks. 'Instead, motherhood is a celebrated part of prominent women's credentials.' Clearly, traditional western society still has a thing or two to learn.

What does all this mean for ordinary pregnant women? Yes, sportswomen are great role models. They have the potential to change society's preconceived ideas around what mothers can achieve; they have the potential to change our own ideas about what we as mums can achieve. But fitness-wise they are on another planet! What have they got to do with the rest of us mums who want to exercise during pregnancy, or afterwards? Mums who stagger their way into the office, school or hospital each morning, who have no time, who are tired? A new report says that only 23 per cent of women exercise when pregnant. After a quick survey of my mum contacts, I'm not surprised. Hardly any of them had been given any meaningful advice from their GP or midwife about how to exercise during pregnancy, or afterwards.

To be clear, this is not about exercising to lose weight; this is about sensible levels of physical activity that equip mums to stay fit and strong in preparation for the later stages of pregnancy, carrying all that extra weight on their skeleton, and then the marathon that is giving birth. Because while I know many mums struggle with their self-esteem during pregnancy, I have to say I found pregnancy liberating in terms of my own body image. After years of worrying what I looked like, I finally felt that my body had a purpose, a function – and it was doing its job brilliantly. When I looked down at my bump, I saw beautiful tightly stretched skin. It was like having my first ever six-pack! A lovely bump, all as it should be. For the first time in my life I was proud of my body. After thirty-two years, it felt like coming home.

What I wasn't prepared for was the medical fear factor. For a start, the only aerobic exercise widely recommended by doctors to pregnant women is swimming. Everything else is deemed unsafe because 'overheating' in pregnancy can cause damage to your unborn child. I don't care how brave you are, that sentence is going to frighten the life out of most mothers, particularly those who might have struggled to conceive, or who have suffered miscarriages. Just that one sentence from a doctor and many mums will give up running, sports and exercise classes on the spot. But what is the definition of overheating? Do they mean sweating? How can we keep fit without sweating? It's making mums more confused than ever. And while swimming is all well and good, and an excellent form of exercise, it's not very convenient. Many women face access issues, and it's so time-consuming, especially prohibitive for mums who already have one or more children. And then there's pool rage, tidal-wave splashing, ignorance of overtaking etiquette, and the general anxiety that so many of us experience when putting our near-naked bodies on display in a swimsuit.

There is walking, of course, as well as pregnancy yoga from twelve weeks, although it tends to cost a bomb and doesn't make you sweat. Or, as my friend Kate put it, 'It's basically relieving women of £10–£15 to lie on the floor humming for an hour.' To be fair, I really loved my pregnancy yoga classes and continued right up to the day I gave birth. I'd recommend any pregnant mum to do them. Although there was an emphasis on relaxation, as Kate describes, alongside that were stretches, posture work, body awareness and important conversations about breathing through birth. I also learned the most useful piece of information anyone told me about giving birth: 'The point where you think you can't continue, where the pain is at its worst, that's transition. You'll think you want to give up, or take drugs, but actually you're nearly there.' That tiny nugget of information was of enormous comfort during my daughter's birth. But the central question of whether or not pregnancy yoga is enough to keep us physically fit through the trimesters, I'm not convinced. And, crucially, neither swimming nor pregnancy yoga seem to be particularly inclusive forms of exercise. When I go swimming, or to a yoga studio, I don't see a great deal of diversity. What are all the other pregnant mums supposed to be doing?

Initially I tried to put on a brave face. I loved my aerobics classes at the local gym, and I'd read online that so long as you had already been doing the exercise before getting pregnant you would be fine to continue. But when I told my aerobics teacher I was pregnant she asked me to leave the class and not return until I had a doctor's note giving me permission to join in. Her words came as a shock. I felt told off, embarrassed and guilty. Did she think I was risking the life of my unborn child with my selfish need for exercise? I never did go back. And that's something I heard again and again: if you fail a woman at any stage of her attempting to play sport or do exercise, she'll rarely have the confidence to go back and try again. Clearly women need more bouncebackability, but maybe the structures around us also need to be more supportive. The result was that I gave up all the fun stuff. I gave up the gym classes I loved, the women I was used to seeing week in, week out, grimacing with over abdominal crunches, and laughing with about complicated step and Zumba routines. After finally finding the joy in exercise, I was now back to exercise as a necessity, not fun.

Despite the GP's warnings, I continued running for the early months of my first pregnancy. With the doctor's words ringing in my head, it felt pretty contraband to run in the park, especially as my bump began to grow. Not to mention the issue of squeezing my sports bra over my newly expanded bust. My husband ran with me, for support and encouragement, and it was hard but it felt good: running along, my little baby inside me, already learning about a healthy life, a pumping heart. I worried, a little, what people might think, seeing my bump bumping along. It's also pretty uncomfortable feeling your bump lollop around, without support. At five months I stopped running. My bump was too big. But I kept swimming and doing pregnancy yoga. It was important to me to do everything I could to be strong and healthy for the birth.

It is, of course, understandable that doctors and midwives would err on the side of caution and warn against doing anything like running, or playing a contact sport. No one wants to tell a pregnant mum that she can carry on with, say, ju-jitsu, only for a fatal blow to the stomach to bring about tragedy to an unborn child. But surely there is more detailed information that medical practitioners can give mothers-to-be? More advice for those who are already active, and more advice for those who want to be? 'Unfortunately, GPs are the same as teachers,' legendary Paralympian Baroness Tanni Grey-Thompson tells me. 'They don't get much help on *how* to prescribe physical activity. Add to that if you're a female GP and you've had a miserable experience of physical activity, you're just going to tell people to walk.'

Tanni says that when she was pregnant with her first child one doctor told her to stop training altogether. She ignored the advice and sought information elsewhere, gleaning it mostly from the Internet, or from contacts in Australia where she believes women are culturally more inclined to be physically active. For Tanni the priority was being able to have a healthy pregnancy, as well as doing everything she could to ensure she was able to compete in the Commonwealth Games six months after her daughter was born.

Tanni is not the only athlete who kept active through her early trimesters. Katie Chapman played football four months into her pregnancy, while Germany and Paris Saint-Germain midfielder Fatmire Alushi played in the 2015 Champions League final well into her second trimester. Topping the bill, though, is the US 800m runner Alysia Montaño who, in 2014, competed at the national championships while eight months pregnant. Sprinting down the final straight, her thirty-four-week-sized bump stuffed into a pink running vest, she was incredible to watch. The fact is that we just don't usually see women with pregnancy bumps physically exerting themselves. It's both shocking and incredibly inspiring. 'I felt such an exhilarating amount of joy,' Alysia said afterwards. 'Having the crowd back me was so unexpected, but I was so excited for it. I was literally laughing out of joy, like, oh my gosh, thank you guys so much!' Even the *Daily Mail* wrote a column in praise of her. Of course Paula Radcliffe famously ran through her pregnancy, while Mary King won team gold and individual bronze at the European Equestrian championships in 1995 when five and a half months pregnant, at a time when pregnancy and sport was a huge taboo.

Former British Olympic team doctor Michael Dooley was one of a close circle of confidants who knew about Mary's pregnancy before it became front- and back-page news. When she revealed her secret to him just weeks away from the European championships she said, 'I'm twenty weeks pregnant, do you mind?'

'Well,' said Michael, 'I was in awe of this woman. I said, "Go for it!"' Michael duly kept her secret for her, and has spent the ensuing twenty years campaigning for more research and guidelines around sport and pregnancy to lessen the taboo. 'That's how I was appointed to the International Olympic Committee to develop guidelines on what to do with a pregnant athlete – because we still don't know! We don't know!' he says, animatedly. 'It's not only what advice to the athlete, it's what advice to the governing bodies? At that time a culture of concealment had developed, which was a nightmare. So I changed the culture to be open about it, I said we mustn't prevent people from competing when they're pregnant, we must develop safe guidelines to help them. That's my philosophy. We've got to make sport safe because exercise is good for you.' There is a caveat though: too much is bad for you, he adds. 'I've just seen an athlete with REDS [Relative Energy Deficiency in Sport, a.k.a. dangerously low body weight] and there are all sorts of associated problems around fertility.'

Michael and I continue to stay in touch over a period of

months. He is one of a number of global experts on a medical advisory group consulting with the IOC on their guidelines for pregnant athletes, due to be published in spring 2016. He is a gold mine of information and I wish I had had a hotline to him when I was first pregnant with my daughter. A fellow of the Royal College of Obstetricians and Gynaecologists (RCOG), Michael co-wrote their guidelines for pregnancy and exercise, and his advice is so much more flexible than anything I have come across elsewhere. For a start, the paper encourages aerobic and strength-conditioning exercise, recommending working at a level that is 'somewhat hard', on a scale from gentle to extremely hard. RCOG advise that exercise does not increase the risk of 'adverse pregnancy or neonatal outcomes', and that moderate exercise does not affect breastfeeding. The only sport banned outright is scuba diving, though there are cautions around horse riding, downhill skiing, gymnastics, ice hockey and cycling because of the risk of falling. Still, existing medical conditions aside, that leaves a huge and joyful scope of exercises that pregnant women can do! Dancing and aerobics and Zumba and running and tennis and badminton and aqua aerobics. Why are none of these mentioned by doctors when pregnant women turn up at their surgeries?

The thing is, if you're an elite athlete, chances are you will have someone like Michael or another highly qualified expert monitoring you. As Tanni told me, 'I had a heart monitor to make sure I wasn't overdoing it, but most women won't have one of those.' So what are the rest of us supposed to do? I wish those RCOG guidelines were more widely distributed, because women desperately need better advice on how to exercise during pregnancy – so that inactive women can be healthier, and so that active women don't overdo it. Unfortunately, that can be the flip side of the equation. One friend of mine, a personal trainer, kept working – which in her case meant some seriously hard running – seven months into her pregnancy, and ended up on crutches in the final weeks before giving birth. Another attended a yoga class so hardcore that the teacher was forcing pregnant mothers into dangerous moves. She also ended up on crutches in the latter stages of her pregnancy and had to hire a nanny to collect her daughter from school because she literally could not manage the short walk. While I stopped running early on in my pregnancy, my job as athletics correspondent was pretty active and I travelled a lot for work. By seven months I was struggling to sit at my desk. My GP referred me to an NHS physio who diagnosed pelvic girdle pain, and gave me various tips on how to tackle it. But working full-time didn't allow for as much rest as I probably needed. On one memorable occasion the pain got so bad I had to lie down in-between paragraphs of a lengthy article and plead for a deadline extension from my editor. We're all at risk of overdoing things, but in terms of medical advice it seems that moderate exercise remains the key to keeping us in the best possible shape throughout our pregnancies. Indeed, Michael mentions a study from Norway which showed that women who exercised before getting pregnant were 14 per cent less likely to suffer from pelvic girdle pain during pregnancy than those who didn't. He also says that moderate exercise will help get you pregnant in the first place – which is a refreshing break from all the mums' message boards that terrorized some of my friends when they were trying for a baby. One friend told me it was all, 'lie down with your legs in the air'; exercise was definitely not on the agenda.

At the end of 2015 two new reports came out about health and pregnancy. A study from Sweden warned mothers not to put on weight in-between pregnancies – even a modest gain of 13lb – as it increased the risk of stillbirth by 30–50 per cent. Another, from Britain's Chief Medical Officer, Sally Davies, urged women to stay fit during pregnancy and not buy into the myth of eating for two. In the latter report, Sally argued that pregnancy was a vital moment of contact between women and the health service, an important opportunity to check in on a woman's overall health, particularly with rising obesity levels (half of all women in the UK aged 25–34 are deemed over-weight). I was thrilled to hear Sally emphasize the role of GPs in advising women on being a healthy weight, and staying physically active. Too often the headlines of these news stories read as yet another example of body-shaming women. It's bad enough that women are told they don't look good, but worse still if we're making women's weight gain responsible for the deaths of babies.

Ultimately, we cannot make this solely a woman's problem. As a society – for the health of future generations – we simply *have* to find a better way to support women to exercise during pregnancy. We have to make antenatal exercise classes more effective – and affordable – limiting us to lying on the floor and breathing is, in itself, not enough. And we have to find a way to give women variety and fun. If women who aren't pregnant struggle to be physically active despite a vast array of sport and exercise on offer, then how can we realistically expect women to engage when we present them with a stultifying choice of swimming, walking and pregnancy yoga? With less than a quarter of women exercising through pregnancy, alarm bells should be ringing. This is a drop-off point where we are potentially losing women from a healthy lifestyle forever. When we talk about a cradle-to-grave approach we must make sure that there isn't a pregnant pause when it comes to pregnancy. The last thing women need is yet another bump in the road.

6

The marathon of motherhood

Just as you nail your pregnancy workout, of course, along comes motherhood. And everything changes all over again. I felt like an alien in those first few days after giving birth. I remember crying inconsolably when my husband popped out to get us a Nando's takeaway because we were too tired to cook. He came back five minutes later with half a chicken and spicy rice, while I sobbed, 'Don't *ever* leave us again, OK?' much to his amusement. I wasn't going mad, it turned out that it was just my milk coming in and yet another flood of hormones to contend with.

The six-week check is every mum's milestone in terms of getting the green light to recommence normal life. It's the moment when mums who had caesareans have their scars checked, and mums with vaginal stitches should be able to stop worrying about what the hell's going on down there. But a 2014 survey of over 4,000 mums, by Netmums and the NCT, found that the six-week check was anything but reassuring. Over 45 per cent felt the check was not thorough enough, and no wonder, with 20 per cent claiming the appointment had lasted less than five minutes. Only 35 per cent were offered an examination of their stitches. The survey did not ask about diastasis recti; unfortunately it is not a check that doctors are obliged to do. But if we are serious about wanting new mums to go back to exercise then surely we need to give them a thorough MOT before we send them out there? As I write, the NHS are undergoing a public consultation about maternity services. But I fear for how conclusive the findings will be. In the online survey, while there are plenty of questions about pregnancy and labour, there is just one tiny box available to comment on your experiences of postnatal care. It shows a worrying lack of priority being given to this area.

If I had my way the six-week check would be offering women so much more. I'd like to see every new mother being checked for diastasis recti, and given advice on simple exercises to solve it. But the reality is that most mums are just not getting the right guidance. My friend Anjana Gadgil, a very active, fit and healthy mum, had a gap as wide as her hand in-between her abdominals. Damningly, it was only diagnosed after her second child. Here is her story:

'When I was three months pregnant with my first child the midwife said, "Oh, your abs have separated already – that's early." I went on to have a second child – again by C-section – and no one, in the many prenatal and postnatal check-ups, ever mentioned it again. So after my second baby, I got to work on my "mummy tummy". Football, tennis, yoga, Pilates, sit-ups. I lost the baby weight but not the tummy. What's more, I had this weird and widening gulf right down the middle of my belly. Finally my sister (a geriatrician) had a look and diagnosed diastasis recti, as she sees it in older people who go on to have hernias.

'My left and right abdominals were five fingers apart, and I was told I would need surgery. My GP had never heard of it. I then stopped all the bad exercise I was doing before. It's not healed but it's a lot better. I have straw-polled many friends and very few know of it, far fewer still how to treat it.'

I find it jaw-dropping that a GP wasn't able to diagnose Anjana, or that countless midwives and health visitors never thought to check for the condition, or mention it. Anjana's story is not an isolated one. During the research for this book I heard more and more horror stories about women with diastasis recti, including one from a woman who lay down in the playground and literally pulled her stomach muscles apart, the gap was so bad. The same story appears repeatedly on Facebook parenting sites, where dozens of women described their experiences. Many had ended up undergoing operations to solve it. Almost no one on the thread had heard of the condition before being diagnosed, often belatedly. Many found their GPs to be clueless and, like Anjana, tried to do sit-ups, planks, crunches and leg raises in an attempt to 'improve' the appearance of their stomach – all of which only made it worse. Surely educating health professionals so that they can diagnose diastasis recti and recommend physiotherapy to remedy it is a far easier and more cost-effective solution than leaving thousands of women to struggle, some of whom end up needing invasive operations paid for by the NHS?

Because diastasis recti is not just about having a 'mummy tummy'. It can cause terrible backache, incontinence and even hernias. One study in the US found that 66 per cent of mums presenting with diastasis recti also had pelvic-floor dysfunction – from incontinence right through to prolapse. Sadly it all seems to be part of a negligent attitude to post-natal health. It is unbelievable to me that in the twenty-first century when a mum says she has backache the response is to shrug, and say it comes with the territory – picking up babies, carrying them in slings, breastfeeding and just general, well, mumness. It is difficult to understand why we can't have doctors, health visitors and midwives checking post-partum mums' abdominals? It takes thirty seconds! And why can't buggyfit instructors, or anyone claiming to specialize in exercise for mums, take five minutes out of each session to do sensible and appropriate core muscle work including the dreaded pelvic-floor exercises that doctors, mothers and grandmothers all constantly tell new mums to do. Women desperately need guidance on how to exercise when there are so many new factors at work in their bodies.

Four years on from my first pregnancy and I have only just found an exercise class that provides that expertise, and I live in London, a city that offers such a variety of experiences that you can even do ballet with your baby – if you're willing to pay £20 a pop. But although my post-baby exercise classes didn't provide the physiological support that I would have liked, they did give me something special. From buggyfit in the park, which taught me the basics of how to push a pram without hurting your body (elbows in, back straight, don't collapse your wrists) and got me out of the house each week, to local community classes for family fitness.

With such scarce provision specifically for post-partum mums, more and more are making their own arrangements. My friend Emmi goes swimming with a group of local mums who take it in turns to watch each other's babies while they do lengths in the pool. Another friend did her own buggy circuits in the park. I also heard about Mothers Meeting, a national movement bringing together mums from the creative industries to have power lunches, 'netwalking' meetups with buggies and Nike workouts, all with their children in tow.

Enter Ready Steady Mums, the brainchild of mum to three small boys Katy Tuncer, and a scheme she has launched in partnership with the Institute of Health Visitors (IHV) to empower mums to get out and exercise. It's true, health visitors don't always have the best reputation with mums: I'll never forget the one who suggested I shave my daughter's hair off at three weeks so that she could have 'nicer hair when she grows up'. I've heard all sorts of moans about contradictory and confusing advice delivered by stern and unapproachable women for whom you instantly regret ever making a cup of tea. But I'm a bona fide cheerleader for Katy's initiative because it's all about bringing mothers together to exercise on their own terms – and using the national institution of health visitors to facilitate it. Currently there are around fifty mum-led groups across the country, but Katy would like to see one set up for each children's centre in the UK – about 3,000. Katy recalls a research paper that found exercise to be the most effective way to support women with mild to moderate postnatal depression, better than antidepressants, and this tallies with RSM's biggest reported benefit of the scheme – increased self-esteem.

'The emotional side is never the ingoing motivation, though,' says Katy of why women sign up to Ready Steady Mums. 'Those tend to be losing the baby weight, and – sadly – mums worrying about being a negative role model to their children, worried about embarrassing their kids by being "fat". Unfortunately we just aren't used to seeing postnatal bodies in the mainstream media, and so even women who felt happy and confident during their pregnancy can feel very differently after they've given birth.' That's something we can all relate to. While it is customary to tell women how great they look in pregnancy, we stop giving them compliments the minute the baby pops out. Katy sends me a link to a project by US photographer Jade Beall, who captured seventy postnatal mums for *A Beautiful Body Project*. The images are extraordinary, and moving. Dimpled stomachs, stretch marks, rounded bodies, breastfeeding boobs. And their lovely children clinging on to them. I stare and stare in amazement. I have never seen women's postnatal bodies made public in this way before. It is a revelation.

What all of these burgeoning initiatives have in common is a set-up where mums can bring their children along with them to exercise, instead of needing to search out crèche facilities or childcare. For me, it is those set-ups that are the most effective, because how many women have the luxury of accessing childcare just so they can exercise? As a new mum I started with buggyfit in the park, which was genius until my daughter reached seven months and decided she hated sitting in a buggy, and, eventually, family fitness at my local Salvation Army branch.

By then Ella was two and learning to socialize. She also wanted to walk more, which meant less buggy time, and less exercise for me. Meanwhile my breastfeeding weight loss had worn off, and I'd developed a tea and cake habit that would make a nutritionist weep. I was short on time and cash, and had run out of childcare favours. Taking Ella to exercise with me at a community centre that charged just £2.50 for an hour was life-changing. It also proved to be a special experience that we could enjoy together. On the good days she would hold my hand and mimic my moves, jogging on the spot, doing star jumps and aerobics grapevines, or sticking her bottom in the air in a comical but cute attempt to do the plank. On the bad days she'd whimper and stretch up her arms for me to cuddle her. I'd star jump with her straddled around my front, laughing at the exertion, and each time peeling her off me and attempting to settle her in the corner with toys and the other children. While I felt the familiar buzz of endorphins, sweat dripping down my temples, my body getting fitter and stronger, she learned how to negotiate toy disputes and foster friendships, exchanging raisins and breadsticks. I loved that time together; it was precious for us and I felt proud as my daughter talked about us doing 'our exercises' and would come home to demonstrate to her dad what we'd been up to. From an early stage in our lives, I felt, we were – both of us – already on the right path to an active lifestyle. At the end of the session volunteers kindly vacuumed up the bread-stick crumbs and squashed raisins, and put away the toys. I felt evangelical about the scheme; I wanted every community centre in the country to have one just like it.

Because while some mums are comfortable, and can afford, to leave their kids at a crèche in the gym, many more will strug-gle with the concept. Whether their children are hard to settle with strangers or are going through periods of separation anxi-ety, or whether the mothers just dread being hauled out of the gym/pool/steam room to soothe their child for the umpteenth time that hour, or simply cannot afford the monthly member-ship fees for a child-friendly gym, a crèche is not the catch-all solution for everyone.

And when we look to elite athlete mums it is interesting how they seem to have reached the same conclusion. Shelley

Rudman, a former skeleton world champion, takes her daughters with her on training camps and homeschools her eldest in-between downhill runs on the ice; eleven times gold-medal-winning Paralympic cyclist Sarah Storey breastfed her daughter Louisa through a return with her, and well into toddlerhood. Like Jessica Ennis-Hill, who often brought Reggie with her or trained at home in a makeshift gym after putting him to bed each night, Sarah always found a way for her daughter to be included in her sessions, whether that was in a Moses basket next to the exercise bike (the whirring noise of the wheels soothing her to sleep), strapped to her torso on a hike across the hillsides, or in the car with husband Barney during her road training sessions. The key to a lot of these set-ups is support. Jess's example speaks volumes. In Toni Minichiello she had a coach who became a parent shortly before she did, and who felt comfortable having a baby around. He understood that her life had changed, that she wouldn't choose between a gold medal and her child, as one ridiculous newspaper headline put it, and that she needed to include Reggie in her day. Crucially, he also understood that everything about her life had changed – from having a new priority in Reggie, to her body facing new and unknown challenges. And he provided the setting to allow her to work quietly through those challenges and find the solutions to regain her strength and sporting prowess. That approach is exemplary. The fact that it paid off in the form of a world championship gold medal shows just how important it is for mums to be supported in their new lifestyle so they can continue to achieve their goals – whether those are world-class sporting performances, or just getting out for a swim with friends.

The more I investigated, the more I discovered that ordinary mums were creating their own mum- and child-friendly exercise environments in their own areas. So, with my daughter in tow, kitted out in exercise gear, I jumped on a train to South London to see my friend and ex Muay Thai fighter Simone Harvey, who runs a boxing class for mums and their children.

Deep in the underbelly of Dulwich Hamlet's football stadium, borrowing the training space used by prize-winning professional boxer Leon McKenzie, a group of women perch on benches outside the men's urinals and tell me their stories. The boxing ring is strewn with toys, while toddlers chat and play and a baby casually chews on a sweaty hand wrap. The women at the class have never met me before, and yet they are so keen to share their stories, to open up about how this class has changed their lives. There's Kate (who I mentioned in the introduction to this book), thirty-nine with two young sons, who had never previously exercised. But two babies later, 'and a hell of a lot of biscuits', her body had changed, and her new form felt unfamiliar and uncomfortable. She didn't like the idea of boxing, but with two kids in tow and childcare to manage, Simone's classes were the only local exercise option to which she could bring her children. 'The first session I was so unfit I only managed to get through the warm-up,' she laughs now. But she was surprised by how quickly she progressed, and soon her husband would come home to find her sparring with Simone in the back garden. Sport and exercise had always been a no-go area for Kate, but in learning to love them, other opportunities began to open in the rest of her life. 'All of a sudden I could do something that I'd always thought was "off limits",' she reflects. 'It's probably no coincidence that I went on to completely rethink my career, taking up an archaeology course at university, something that I'd wanted to do my whole life but had always been discouraged from pursuing. My dad had said it wasn't a suitable job for women.' Kate is now studying for an MSc in Palaeolithic archaeology.

Anna, thirty-six, with two children, has a similar story. Originally a solicitor, she retrained as a video artist. Before attending Simone's classes she'd always hated sport, though not exercise, and particularly the idea of anything to do with boxing. 'People kept posting on the parents' forum about a local boxing class. I thought, "How hilarious, I'm never going to do that!"' Whenever her husband watched boxing on the TV Anna would leave the room; she says it made her feel physically sick. But after five years of pregnancy, childbirth, breastfeeding, childcare, she felt ready for a different physical challenge – importantly, one that could sit alongside motherhood. 'I wanted to re-engage with my own physicality, for myself. It's not that I needed "me time", or something different to the kids. But my children had reached an age where my body wasn't being used solely for them anymore. I wanted to explore how my body could be enjoyed in a different way.' Anna took up running and started a dance class, but the boxing had a unique attraction to it – on at the right time for the kids' routines, and best of all she could bring her youngest with her. 'I know people say you can use a crèche at a gym, but that's never appealed to me. I really want to know who's looking after my children.'

When Anna tells me she is pregnant with her third child I can't help feeling a bit shocked. I've just done several rounds punching pads, and then holding pads for another woman to punch at me. My doctor's warning haunts me – is it really safe to be pregnant in a boxing gym? Anna explains. 'I wouldn't walk into any old boxing gym and let them punch at me, but this is a special environment, just for mums, where everyone's looking after one another, and we've all been through the same thing. The precaution I take is going to a class where it's run by a mum, for mums. I wouldn't tell every mother to run out and join a boxing class – I don't want to pile pressure on anyone to be active – but for me personally it is important to be fit and strong to carry this child, and to be healthy when I give birth.' Through the drills Anna is careful to hold her pad away from her body, rather than close to her abdomen, so that her sparring partner is not punching directly at her. The atmosphere is supportive and encouraging, Simone keeps a watchful eye and everyone is alert to the babies crawling on the floor, toddlers waddling around the gym and mothers breastfeeding in the corner.

Isobel, twenty-seven, an interiors and murals specialist with two young sons, drives an hour into London each week just to attend the class. Her kids love it, knocking about the boxing ring with the other toddlers and a sea of toys, and she loves the can-do atmosphere of mums sweating it out in a gritty gym. 'I love doing a form of exercise that makes you think,' she says. 'I do feel like my mind is rotting a little bit with children; as much as I try and engage them with things, it's not as intellectually stimulating. Learning new things is good for my brain.' As Simone shouts out each new pads routine – *CROSS, LEFT HOOK, UPPER CUT, LEFT HOOK, CROSS!* – I can see what she means about having to stay alert.

When Isobel had her first son she was twenty-four years old, and the youngest mum in her NCT class. 'I was at university studying at the time. I finished my degree on the Friday and had Stanley on the Monday. I was the first of my friends to have kids.' Despite her age, after two large babies, she felt Mother Nature had given her an unfair deal. 'I seemed to end up with the worst body and scars out of all of them. I've got horrendous stretch marks and sagging skin all over my stomach and my boobs. I'm fitter and skinnier than I've ever been but I still have a blimmin' turkey stomach hanging off me, honestly, it's dreadful, I can't seem to get rid of it. I didn't realize I was that vain but pregnancy really took its toll on my body, it had an effect far greater than just physically.' To me Isobel looks amazing. She's tall and strong with well-defined shoulders; she looks like an athlete. And she's got the coolest bleached crew cut I think I've ever seen on a mum. Despite her body hang-ups, it's clear just how much she gets from exercising. She runs several times a week. 'It's the only time I get twenty minutes away from the kids,' she laughs. 'I know that sounds awful! But it feels like a relief, a place to clear to my mind.'

Every mother I know says that about exercise. It's a space for yourself. A very modern room of one's own, in a disconnected virtual age where we need to connect to our bodies more than ever. But creating that space can seem impossible. Whether it's housework, bedtimes, school pickups or trying to maintain a social life, mothers are constantly negotiating their schedules, with partners, childcare providers, employers. Negotiating yet another element – exercise – can seem the very last straw. We know that if only we would get out there and do it we would feel great, but still it languishes, the item at the very bottom of the list, down there with tax returns and cleaning the skirting boards. When I think about the men I know in my life, they don't seem to have this problem. They announce, 'I'm going to the gym,' or 'I'm going to play football.' It's not a point of negotiation, unless there's a specific practical reason why they can't go. This is a great template, mothers! Exercise shouldn't be a point of negotiation, it's your health, your sanity, your time and space. You can do it with friends as part of socializing, or you can do it on your own. And I hope you will also be able to do it with your kids. The more avenues we can offer women to be physically active, the better.

The problem is that it's so easy to fall off the wagon when you've got children. You do buggyfit, and then they decide they hate their buggy. You go to aerobics, and they get separation anxiety. You do classes together on a weekday morning, and then your child starts nursery.

When I fell pregnant for the second time I had pretty much stopped exercising. Everything had fallen by the wayside, and the new routine of pickups and drop-offs at nursery and attempting to squeeze a career in between filled my days. I knew this wasn't a good state of affairs, but I couldn't figure out how to change things. My husband bought me a beautiful pair of deep-purple running shoes and a luxury sports bra, but the trainers sat in the hallway for several months and the sports bra remained neatly folded in its pretty box.

I thought back to my first pregnancy and how I used to go running through the park, but things were different this time around. I already had a child to look after, and three part-time jobs to squeeze into three and a half days a week. And I felt so sick; when my daughter had her bath I lay on my side on the hallway landing fighting the nausea.

Twelve weeks arrived. But as the date of our first scan drew closer, something unexpected happened. A tiny spot of blood appeared. It was unremarkable, really, so miniscule I could easily have missed it. But it was definitely pink, definitely blood.

I ignored it. The next day there was a bigger drop. And then another. On the third day there was more still. I called the NHS helpline; they said to go to A & E, but that in all likelihood it was nothing. Light bleeding is very common in early pregnancy and usually nothing to worry about. My husband flew to Portugal; I told him everything would be fine.

The following morning something was definitely wrong. I started to cry, and my daughter climbed into my lap. 'I just need to check everything's OK with the baby,' I told her, trying to sound calm. 'We'll go to hospital, just to make sure.' In A & E we sat on cold grey chairs, with my parents. My dad bought crisps and grapes for the wait. I hoped no one with scary-looking injuries would walk into reception and frighten my daughter.

There are layers to an accident and emergency admission. You have to patiently go through them, retelling your story at each point, before you get to the person who can actually diagnose what is happening to your body. Until that happens, there is nothing to do but wait. Eventually my daughter got bored. I'd never been so pleased to hear her say those words. I packed her off to the park with my dad, and hunkered down in my chair.

Two hours later my mum and I finally reached the emergency gynaecological unit. The doctor scanned my belly, twisting and prodding with the probe, pulling together a picture on a screen that I could not see. Suddenly she stopped. 'I'm going to need to do an internal scan, the baby looks very small,' she said.

'Is that your mum in the waiting area?' I nodded. 'I think she'd better come in.'

Sitting beside me in the half-light, my mum held my hand. The tears began to flow. Would my baby be OK? There were only two possible answers: yes, and no. Inside my head I battled between the extremes. Should I steel myself for the worst? Or hope for the best?

It felt like a long time, lying in that semi-darkness, waiting to hear. Eventually the doctor removed the probe, hung it up in its socket, and folded her hands in her lap. She turned her face towards me, with solemn lips. 'It's not good news, I'm afraid,' she said. The baby had stopped growing. It was very small. 'No one knows why these things happen. You can take a moment to get dressed, and then we will need to talk about how to remove it.'

You cannot imagine how fast that transition is, between hearing that your baby is dead, and being told you must now decide how to get rid of it. I got dressed and we sat in chairs, holding leaflets, listening, trying to understand. There are five options: tablets at home, tablets at hospital, an operation under general anaesthetic, an operation under local anaesthetic. Or you can leave it to Mother Nature to do the job for you, but effectively that means walking around with a dead foetus inside your womb for an unquantifiable length of time.

I forced myself to make the decision. I would have the operation. It was the quickest solution, and I needed to be well again for my daughter. I rang my husband. Far away on the other end of the phone he tried to be my support. He had packed his bags already; he was on his way to the airport; he'd sit in departures until they let him take a flight home.

We wandered out into the daylight, my mum and I, adjusting to the light. A busy street market was on across the road. Plastic bowls of brightly coloured bird's-eye chillis sat alongside piles of bitter karela and mountains of fresh herbs. Everywhere we looked there were crates of pale-orange Alfonso mangoes, the sweetest and most fragrant you can buy. We took half a dozen, and went home.

My husband came home late that night, exhausted. But home. We all piled into our bed, our daughter snoring gently between us; we held hands over her. There would be a few days to wait until the operation, we just had to rest.

But nature had its own ideas. Two days later my body began to bleed heavily. Lumps falling out of me. I always assumed when someone had a miscarriage that there was a body. Sometimes there is, but I just had lumps. What can you do with lumps? They are nothing to say goodbye to, to cry over. They came steadily, like ripe plums slowly falling out of a tree.

My daughter asked me where the baby was. It was a good question. I didn't know the answer. In the language of the hospital there was no baby, there was 'blood' and there was 'tissue'. But an unborn baby is more than the sum of its parts. In that baby is vested the hopes and dreams of a family, the excitement, the planning, the worry, the love. Things that leap into life long before an egg is even fertilized by a sperm. My daughter had been planning on becoming a big sister; she was proud and excited, she wanted to hold our baby, tickle it, feed it and rock it to sleep. Now where had it gone? I struggled to explain.

By the day of the operation I was convinced it had all come out. My husband helped me to the hospital, and I painstakingly climbed the stairs on the Tube, surreally floating through the rush hour with tiny close-legged steps, trying not to let anything more fall out.

At the EGU they scanned me again, blood dripping freely on the floor this time as I lay on the bed. I glanced down: the grey lino looked like something out of a horror movie. I grimaced. Thank goodness for the chirpy NHS nurse who had done this job for thirty years; she'd seen it all before. She'd fetch me a tea, and a nice chocolate bourbon.

Until then I sat in a recovery room. Not everything had come out. The nurses were going to bring me some tablets. Five tiny blue ones, three white ones. Take them all, then wait. My body began to shiver, then burn. The room spun. I felt scared and weak. The contractions began; I knew this pain, I'd felt it before. But last time I was standing in a sunny room, at the start of a journey that would end with our beautiful daughter in my arms. The end of this journey would deliver no such joy. I laboured and squeezed my husband's hand. At the end of this, I said in-between painful contractions, we will go on an amazing holiday. He smiled. Wherever you want to go, we'll do it, he promised. The nurses were wonderful. Somehow, slowly, I began to recover. I sipped at a cup of overly sugared tea, and managed half the chocolate bourbon. 'You look so much better now,' beamed the doctor.

What has a miscarriage got to do with sport and exercise? Well, this book is the story of a woman's body – not just mine, all of ours. And the things that happen to our bodies connect and disconnect us from sport and exercise throughout our lives. Pregnancy, childbirth, miscarriages, breastfeeding, abortions, menstruation and the menopause: these are all processes that so many women encounter at some point in their lives. They are the common traumas of the female body, and yet we remain silent about them, reinforcing our own *omertà*. And in that silence grows myth, and misunderstanding, ignorance, anxiety and confusion. In the process of researching this book I heard over and over again from medics how women do not know their own bodies. Mr Dooley says he speaks to high-powered, intelligent women who don't understand the basics of their own reproductive health, while an article in the *Guardian* revealed how another doctor had been asked by a mother of four what a 'uterus' was.[27] Certainly, most of the time, we don't even know how to refer to our reproductive organs. But if we don't know our own bodies, that's because we are not encouraged to talk about them – from the young woman who posted a picture of her menstrual blood on Instagram only to be greeted by death threats, to the universal absence of periods, childbirth and miscarriages in mainstream media. One in five women suffers a miscarriage, and yet their stories are rarely told.

And yet as my own story clumsily tumbled out, I was overcome by the number of people – men and women – who told me about losing their babies. Friends, neighbours, colleagues, family of friends, mothers, daughters, dads: they all shared their stories, unprompted. Over the garden wall, at the nursery gate, in Tube carriages, through text messages and transatlantic phone calls. So many stories, whispered, clandestinely shared. There were double losses, quadruple losses, losses that made some give up, and losses that emboldened others to keep trying. There were losses in the early weeks, and losses midway through, women delivering their lost foetus through labour. And, perhaps saddest of all, the loss of a full-term baby, a stillborn, bringing tears to all.

As I lay in bed wondering how to explain to colleagues and friends that I would have to cancel commitments for the rest of the week, I felt a strange sense of debilitation. And an overwhelming urge to move. Now that I was being ordered to rest, I was desperate to be active.

I waited two weeks for the all-clear, and then, one sunny morning, set off to the park with my box-fresh trainers and sports bra for my first run in four years. It felt like liberation. Running for my body, running for my life. Running for me. It hurt like hell, of course. My lungs ached, my heart was unused to the pulse. I wanted to stop; everything felt uncomfortable, and I felt self-conscious, my stomach still swollen from what had been growing in there for so many weeks before. But I also felt pretty amazing. Walking back home, my brain was levitating somewhere just above my head, enjoying the early-summer breeze. I felt the power in my legs, striding along, buzzing off the endorphins. For the next six weeks I ran regularly, getting stronger, and loving it.

That's how I rediscovered exercise. As a mum I have loved and lost my relationship with exercise countless times. All those interruptions – the baby that grows too big to sit patiently for buggyfit, then starts crawling, then walking, then running; the separation anxiety that stops you leaving your child for any more time than you need to; the new childcare arrangements; using up every childcare favour under the sun; the increasing hours at work. Each and every time you have to make a new adjustment, up your game, reinvent yourself, start afresh. It's exhausting.

And all the while we're raising our daughters and sons to repeat the same mistakes, the same stereotypes. Because we don't know how to play football in the park together, we're rubbish at throwing them the ball, we rarely sprint down the road together just for fun, and we don't encourage them to watch sport. Life cycle, déjà vu.

As Michelle Obama observed, mums are fundamental in changing the status quo for the next generation, as well as ourselves. The First Lady made a crucial link between mums and exercise, and why that connection is so very important. Because it's not just about being healthy, it's about being a role model, and making time for yourself as a woman. And how many mums do you know who do that? 'When I get up and work out, I'm working out just as much for my girls as I am for me,' says Michelle Obama, 'because I want them to see a mother who loves them dearly, who invests in them, but who also invests in herself. It's just as much about letting them know that as young women it is OK to put yourself a little higher on your priority list.' Michelle Obama's campaign to end childhood obesity in America manages to show us why, for women, being physically active is a feminist statement. And she still looks cool at fifty slam-dunking LeBron James in the White House.

One of the mums I met at Simone's boxing class has a simple story that sticks in my head. Her name is Jess, a twenty-nine-year-old nurse from South London, who started exercising again while she was still breastfeeding her second child. Jess was able to go to the class because Simone adapted the exercises around her feeding needs. No other class worked for her – she felt she couldn't leave her daughter in a crèche – and with a toddler son she was excluded from mother-and-baby exercise classes or buggyfit, which is geared towards one child in a pram. Jess reminds me a bit of Jessica Ennis-Hill: that same naturally athletic physique, a glowing fitness. I assume she'll tell me she always loved sport, but instead she surprises me and says she hated PE at school. Thankfully for Jess, she had amazing role models in her parents, who both went running every week. 'My brother did too. That's probably why I did. It just seemed normal.'

Those four simple words are so precious. They are what we surely want every girl and woman to feel. To feel normal. To feel comfortable doing something physically active. And that's where mums come in. Because every time we exercise we are inadvertently showing our children a pathway to a brighter future.

Sometimes we don't even know how bright. Take the example of Olympic champion cyclist Laura Trott, who took up the sport because of her mum. Glenda Trott was a size 24 before she started cycling, but being denied entry to a cable-car ride while on holiday with her family in the US prompted her to make a drastic change. Her doctor advised her to start swimming, but she couldn't bear the thought of braving a public pool and so she bought a bike instead, and began training at the local track in Welwyn Garden City. The whole family went with her. 'Mum wasn't sporty and then all of a sudden she turned into superwoman,' Trott said in an interview with the *Telegraph*. 'She'd be on the indoor trainer before work; she'd cycle ten miles in the afternoon with her friends and then when my dad came home from work she'd go out with him, too.'[28] Glenda lost eight and a half stone in eighteen months. Little did she know that both of her daughters would become obsessed with cycling, or that Laura would go on to become one of Britain's most decorated riders.

The thing is, if Glenda hadn't been brave enough to get on a bike, or hadn't had the support of her family to cycle with her, none of this might ever have happened. All these years later, Glenda could still be back at her local doctor's surgery, upset about her weight, crash-dieting, refusing to go to the pool. Glenda says she put on the weight after having her children, like so many women. It is crucial that we start supporting mums at this critical point in their lives, and supporting them in the right way. It could change the lives of millions of mothers, and it could change the futures of millions of children. And, who knows, we might even produce a few more Olympic champions along the way.

7

'Are you the tea lady?'
and other common questions

It's never pretty, arriving at a press box to write a match report if you're late. All the other journos are already assembled, packed in together, a musty smell of old jumpers. If curry's been served as the pre-match meal, there will be at least one colleague with an irritable bowel. Noting your seat number – bugger, it's right in the middle of the row – you inch your way along, as one after another of Her Majesty's press pack reluctantly stands up to let you past. In the narrow space you do your very best to avoid all contact with genital areas. A quick scramble around the floor to find a plug socket for your laptop, and, crouching down, you think you're finally home and dry. Just then you hear a voice. It's coming from the bloke sitting next to you, who's old enough to be your dad. 'While you're down there, love . . .' he says, his smut-filled grin prompting giggles from the surrounding seats. Cue face-burn, and ninety minutes of disbelief. Welcome to the male-dominated world of sports journalism, a place that I have called home for the last twelve years.

On meeting MediaCom's Sue Unerman for this book, I

relayed the same anecdote to her and she laughed knowingly. 'But what did he mean?' I ask. 'He can't really have meant, y'know? Did he?' She gives me a look. 'Haven't you heard that one before?' she asks. 'That's a classic; I've heard it so many times, and yes, that's exactly what they mean.' I realize I've spent the best part of a decade giving this guy the benefit of the doubt. Because I just can't fathom why anyone would make a joke about fellatio in a professional situation with a woman they had only just met.

It wasn't to be my only encounter. Sure enough, over the years, I heard many other jokes like these, as have so many female colleagues in the sports industry. But what do you say if someone makes such a disgusting joke? No one wants to make a fuss. No one wants to be that victim. No one wants to spoil the party, even if the party isn't feeling very fun, and you're not sure you actually want to be there at all. In defence of 'while you're down there love', he was probably still shell-shocked to meet a woman in his world. Yes, there are also plenty of examples of supportive male colleagues, but it is hard to ignore the fact that every woman I know who works in sport – or even just likes it – routinely gets asked if they're in the right place: 'Are you the tea lady, love?' 'Are you waiting for your boyfriend?' 'Do you actually like sport, then?' Because whether you are a woman working in the sports industry, or simply a female sports fan switching on the telly, the two are not generally expected to mix. Women are accepted as titillating accessories to the sporting action – but as fans? Or journalists? Or match officials? Or CEOs? Not so much.

As British Formula One driver and playboy Jenson Button famously put it, breasts and periods get in the way of sport.

According to him, women and sport are biologically incompatible. 'One week of the month you wouldn't want to be on the circuit with [women], would you?' he told *FHM* in 2005. 'A girl with big boobs would never be comfortable in the car. And the mechanics wouldn't concentrate. Can you imagine strapping her in?' Bizarrely, I can't seem to find any instance of Jenson complaining about the Grid Girls.

And that's because female totty is seen as so wholly appropriate in sport that we hardly bat an eyelid as TV cameras pan across a sports crowd, searching for a hottie. From Wimbledon to the World Cup, it's the same story. The underlying message to the viewer is that sport on TV replicates the male heterosexual gaze. If you're a woman watching you're simply an anomaly. The trend launched the career of one of the twentieth century's biggest-ever sex symbols: Pamela Anderson, spotted in the crowd by TV cameras at a Canadian Football League game in the 1980s. Meanwhile, cheerleaders account for the most prominent female figures across much of US men's team sport. Then there's the 'pit girls' employed to stand about in hot pants with zippable cleavage, holding umbrellas for motor-sport drivers, and ring girls at boxing bouts holding up cards to tell us the number of the next round. Recently, watching Chris Eubank's son's fight on TV, I stared in disbelief as the presenter apologized for Chris saying 'cojones' on air. Why is that word deemed offensive when employing half-naked women as objects to stare at is not? And if scantily clad ladies are all just a harmless bit of fun, then why – at my first-ever boxing match, Amir Khan's professional debut – did the crowd around me talk about those women with such sexual aggression? 'Phwoar, look at her!' one of them started up. 'I'd let her piss on my face any day.' I literally wanted to crawl under my seat.

Even women's sport is not immune. At the Flanders Diamond tour during the summer of 2015 four women in tiny bikinis flanked the winners on stage, much to the chagrin of Dutch cyclist Marijn de Vries, who boldly highlighted the issue on Twitter. Brilliantly, US cyclist Anna Zivarts photoshopped some men in Speedos onto pictures of Chris Froome on the podium to ram home the point, and the Belgian organizers apologized for the incident. But the bigger question is: why, in the twenty-first century, does sport need to be sexualized at all?

I'm not convinced that sport has woken up to this as a discussion point. It remains a blind spot. Take cycling's global governing body, UCI, getting worked up about a women's team whose kit accidentally made them appear naked from the waist down. The Colombia Bogotá Humana kit included a strip of flesh-coloured fabric across the midriff which, when photographed in a certain light, looked a bit camel-toe. The images sent the UCI into comic meltdown, with president Brian Cookson labelling it 'unacceptable by any standard of decency'. The double messaging here is incredible: it is OK to have models in skimpy bikinis on the winners' podiums, but if it looks too much like the real thing – albeit innocently, and accidentally – then it is a sign of abhorrent indecency.

I'm often asked if one sport is worse than another. I'm not convinced it's helpful to compare, and in any case frustrating stories seem to come to light in every sport I've come across. People inevitably argue that sport is merely a reflection of wider societal attitudes. True, to some extent. But if we leave the conversation there then we also leave sport with a get-out-of-jail card, the shrug of the shoulders, 'what can anyone actually do?' approach. That frustrates me. There's *so* much we can do to change things. In *Do It Like A Woman*, a book about women changing the world, Caroline Criado-Perez explored the full spectrum of feminism and sexism, so I ask her whether sport is different from any other sector. Her response is illuminating. 'Well, I suppose the same preconceptions and prejudices that discriminate against women in one field is the same in another,' she nods, 'but I guess with sport there's something about the way women aren't encouraged to be active, the way women are constantly represented as passive. It's like in films where women are less likely to have the main role, and instead be in a supporting role, often getting in the way of the hero doing his thing. Sport is such an obvious manifestation of that in the way that women are not encouraged to be active.' And there's the irony. In sport, the most physically active of sectors, we routinely reduce women to the most passive, nonspeaking roles. When women dare to play a speaking part – a journalist, a manager, a chief executive – or an active part – a player, a referee, a medic – they are going against the grain. And it grates.

Caroline believes this trend is key to preventing women from genuinely engaging in sport and exercise. Of course it is. From the very start we are limiting girls' aspirations as to how they can get involved in sport. They are shown only marginal roles that rely on being conventionally sexy or pretty. Meanwhile boys in sport can look any way they like: no one cares. They are judged solely on their talent.

This is the crux of the problem when it comes to getting women and girls physically active. The mainstream media perpetuates the notion that women should focus entirely on a static image of a perfect body as the end goal. There are no messages about the process, the active body, how it makes us feel in that moment. 'That's what I think is really missing from how sport and exercise is presented to women,' says Caroline. 'It's not about being able to do really fucking cool shit with your body, it's about do I look good in a bikini? And that's just not inspiring! It doesn't make you want to do it. So when you're actually exercising all you're thinking is, "At the end will I have a nice body?", not, "Look at my fucking legs go as I'm running!" which actually keeps you running, and even changes the way you do the exercise. I enjoy it more when I think, "Wow, I just did that sprint, that's awesome," instead of, "If I do this two times a week, by the end of the summer I won't have a massive belly." I think we're really missing a trick in terms of how we're presenting it to women. Especially for women it's something that's so little offered to us, the opportunity to think of ourselves as powerful and strong and capable, that our bodies are tools. It's kind of intoxicating.'

To me, that's a reason in itself to recognize the This Girl Can campaign as groundbreaking. Prior to its launch we had never before seen images of women being physically active on mainstream TV in that way, in prime-time advertising slots. We had never been encouraged to enjoy the movement of our bodies just as they are, without reference to whether they look good or not, or whether they are on their way to losing any weight. But watching Sport England's campaign advert we are shown the joy and determination on the women's faces. We see the process, not the end result. It's a powerful message that goes against the grain of pretty much every single mainstream media campaign depicting women's bodies.

For Caroline, the strength part of the equation has been key. She rediscovered sport at the age of thirty after a friend wrote a blog about getting physically strong. 'It was the first time I'd read anything like that,' she says now. 'Usually when women write about their body it's always about how they hate it; only men write about getting strong.' Inspired, she joined a gym and started lifting weights, enjoying the satisfaction of being able to measure her progress through the amount of weight she could lift. Boxing, running and climbing came into the picture and soon she was 'addicted'. For the most part, men have been supportive; she says it's those that are insecure, perhaps less confident in their own abilities – like the men who sent her death and rape threats around her Bank of England campaign – who get huffy, who roll their eyes or sigh impatiently as she lifts. But exercising in a public space does attract unwanted attention, and she worries particularly for younger women who may be put off by the intimidation. 'Sometimes, I'll box in the park with a female friend and you will get men who clearly have not boxed a day in their lives running up to you and telling you you're doing it all wrong! It's that sense of, "This is a male domain, and I have a sense of entitlement over it." And that happens quite a lot. Men want to show they know more about this than you do. Guys who heckle and catcall. It's fine for me as I'm old enough and feminist enough that it doesn't affect me, but if I was younger I would probably feel less secure and stop doing it. What I find really interesting is that every woman I tell about my boxing says, 'Oh my God, that's so cool, can I come with you?' I think there's that untapped desire among women to be strong and be able to defend themselves and have a skill.'

I wonder about this. As a young girl I remember wanting to be able to skateboard like the boys in my class. I also wanted to learn to juggle, to do wheelies on a bike, and I dreamed about how cool it would be to be able to run rings around the boys in the playground with a football. I never achieved any of those things. If I'm honest, I didn't truly dare to. And so, as the teenage years quickly set in, I left those ambitions behind. It didn't seem necessary to have those physical skills any more. But if I cast my mind back I can still remember the absolute thrill I felt daydreaming about how brilliant it would be to pull off any number of those tricks. When I think about the men I know, and the sheer pleasure they still get from doing something impressive in a game of five-a-side football, or artfully skimming a stone across water, I can't help but feel envious. They still have that physical, playful element in their lives. And it makes them happy. Wouldn't it be great if women and girls could have this too?

Imagining Caroline in the park, sparring with a friend, I'm reminded of a phone call with my mum. Out of the blue she told me that she'd seen a woman boxing in her local park and she really liked the look of it. She liked the idea of being strong. This is my seventy-one-year-old mum who has never done sport in her life, outside of swimming, yoga and walking. I think about women doing these things in public spaces and how very powerful that is. How far that idea can radiate. In going out there and actually doing it, we give others permission to try it for themselves. We make it easier to change the status quo.

But to be the person who stands out, who makes the difference, is not always easy. Annie Zaidi is a young coach from Coventry making waves in the football industry. As a woman, and as an hijab-wearing Muslim, the expectation is that she should be working with Muslim women, or coaching women's football. Annie, though, is clear about which direction she wants to take. She doesn't wish to be pigeonholed; she's got her eye on a role in professional men's football, and though it's early days in her career she's already starting to make an impact – working at QPR with Les Ferdinand and Chris Ramsey. I've met Annie quite a few times. She's a huge character – talking about taking over from Arsène Wenger and fancying Thierry Henry. She's feisty and jokey and outspoken and full of laughs. But when she agrees to be interviewed for this book I hear about another side of her, a young woman who has overcome extreme barriers in her life. I listen, spellbound, as she tells me her story.

Growing up, Annie suffered from chronic eczema; she was in and out of hospital for weeks on end, covered in bandages. When the condition flared up, she says, you could hardly make out her eyes. She missed a lot of school, and was bullied for it. 'People judge you on how you look,' she says. 'I've had suitors who refused me because of my eczema. Football became my escape from all the bullshit. I'd pull a hoodie over my face, and football was my best friend.' But it wasn't quite as simple as that. In organized football Annie was expected to wear shorts, which exposed her skin to grass and made her eczema worse. Then there was the routine of a traditional Muslim Pakistani background, attending mosque five days a week after school, and cooking with her mum on Saturdays. 'I may not know how to do a Cruyff turn, but I can cook a killer chicken biryani,' she laughs. The community didn't like her wearing tracksuit bottoms – 'man clothes' – it wasn't becoming for an Asian girl. 'My mum's been my biggest fan, she accepts what I do, but it's hard to change generations, to change cultures.'

As Annie tried to pursue a coaching career, she faced prejudice at every turn. There were those in her own community who called her 'coconut' or 'Bounty', the Muslim cleric who crossed the road to tell her she was a bad role model, and the racial slurs from white girls. And everyone had an opinion about which direction her coaching should take: some said she should coach Muslim girls only; meanwhile after the 7/7 terrorist attacks in London, a local Muslim football club said her hijab would be off-putting to prospective parents worried about Islamophobia and extremism. Annie finally found a role coaching an under-elevens boys' team. Out of 400 managers, she was the only female. On the touchline she experienced sexist and racist abuse from opposition managers and parents. If she complained, she was seen as a troublemaker. 'You've got to have a thick skin to work in football,' she says, 'but even so I had to leave that job because it was poisoning my love for the game.' She told her mum about the abuse. 'My mum joked, "What do you expect? It's a man's world! It's like your dad coming into the kitchen and messing things up!"' Annie laughs.

But she couldn't leave coaching behind altogether; it was too important. 'At one point I was working with victims of sexual exploitation as part of a youth community role in the West Midlands. They were from all races, and they'd never played football before. One of the girls said to me, "This is the first time I've ever felt empowered in my life." I knew what she meant. The moment a football touches the soles of my feet, something comes over me. I feel protected and safe.' I tell Annie what a powerful image she paints. She nods, sagely. 'Well, I'm talking about the soles of my feet, but I'm also talking about my soul. It's both.'

Annie's message of empowerment through sport is vital for all girls to hear. I want to send her into schools with a megaphone, spreading the word. There is something intensely therapeutic about simply playing with a ball, having a run, focusing on something physical. As a modern society we are obsessed with achieving this kind of mental state – there are even mindfulness and Zen colouring books – but how amazing if we could just give everyone a ball to play with?

Annie says she is lucky enough to have been mentored by some amazing men and women who want to see her succeed: Chris Ramsey, Les Ferdinand, Wallace Hermit (who co-founded the Black and Asian Coaches' Association), and England Women's assistant manager Marieanne Spacey. But there are those who do her down, or tell her she's a tick box and that's the only reason why she gets opportunities. She faces a dilemma that all women can relate to – should we tell our stories? Reveal our challenges? Speak out against prejudice, and risk being cast as the victim? Or do we keep quiet and soldier on, leaving others to wonder forever if they are the only ones who experience this stuff? Personally, I respect Annie for sharing her experiences, for telling it like it is, for standing up for what she believes in. I don't see her as a victim; I see her as a strong woman, leading the way for others, making their paths that little bit easier. 'Women need other women,' Annie says plainly. 'It's good getting support from the men, but they don't go through the BS we go through as women. Women are a team, we support each other, and women in football have been my greatest teammates, my left back and right back, my centre forwards and centre halves.'

This is exactly why Women in Football came about, the network of women employed in the football industry that I co-founded with Shelley Alexander in 2006. We exist to give other women a voice when they don't always feel they can speak out. Or to back them when they do. We exist to tell the football industry that women should not be sexually harassed in the workplace, or sacked because they've had a child, or paid less, or talked down to, or denied job opportunities, or subjected to comments about being a lesbian, or asked to hoover the carpet or serve tea in the boardroom instead of doing the roles they are qualified to do. Over the years women have come forward to tell us about their experiences in the industry – and we have been horrified by the abuse they have faced, and amazed at their incredible stoicism.

Because while there have been high-profile male-orientated campaigns around racism and homophobia in football – which has helped to improve the atmosphere at many football grounds – incredibly, nothing significant has ever been done to tackle sexism in the stands. Women make up 51 per cent of the national population, and 25 per cent of the Premier League match day revenue. If for no other reason than pure economics, why would you ignore half the population by not including sexism in the equality equation?

Sometimes I wonder whether football even understands the basics of sexism. Having a conversation about sexism with the football authorities is often like banging your head against a wall. While other industries – including construction – have been forced to change their ways, football is still holding on to an idea of life that belongs in the 1970s. And so while my local police force recently encouraged women to call if they experience harassment on the street such as catcalling or wolf-whistling, football says it can do nothing about thousands of fans wolf-whistling a female medic running onto a pitch to assist an injured player. And it's not just wolf whistles. Chants can range from the ubiquitous 'She's a whore,' to 'Get back in the kitchen,' 'Tits and fanny,' and 'Does she take it up the arse?' TV presenter Gabby Logan was a well-known recipient of 'Get your tits out for the lads,' though her blushes were spared when Sir Bobby Charlton gallantly got his out and jiggled them about a bit. If only we all had an England World Cup-winning legend in our corner.

Sometimes the abuse takes on a darker tone. If you're a Coventry fan you may remember the chants commemorating striker Marlon King's conviction for sexual assault: 'She said yes, Marlon,' and 'She's a ho, Marlon.' Then there's the section of Sheffield United fans who sang 'She's a whore,' about the woman who was raped by footballer Ched Evans. Or simply, 'He shags who he wants.' Or the Arsenal fans who vented their frustration at Robin Van Persie's move to Manchester United by referencing his arrest for rape in 2005 (sung to the tune of Craig David's 'Rewind'): 'Van Per-sie, when a girl says no – molest her.' Inevitably the fans' forums frequently brush off all this stuff as 'banter', advising 'If you don't like it, don't come to football' – a line that would rarely now be considered an adequate response to racism. But these are not isolated incidents. One season ticket holder told me about a man shouting, 'When I get home the wife's going to get a fucking kicking,' because their team had lost. A TV reporter had to endure the word 'slut' being chanted at her during a live broadcast. And former Chelsea doctor Eva Carneiro was roundly abused by opposition fans during the 2014/15 season, with comments such as, 'Show us where you piss from, you slag.' The clubs responsible faced no sanctions from the governing bodies.

The age-old defence for this stuff is that football is a sport for working-class men to enjoy. The one day of the week they get to relax. They've paid for their seat, they should be able to shout whatever they want. And anyway, it's all just a laugh. But football, to its credit, is evolving beyond that. It has rejected the hooligan-tarred image of fans from the 1980s, and instead embraced community schemes and family enclosures. The sport is starting to make the right noises about being inclusive. But there remains a long way to go yet.

Even if you take away the overtly offensive stuff, you're still left with a lot of assumptive football songs where men are the default and it's uncomfortable to join in if you're female. A quick survey of my football-going female friends revealed that most of them don't sing the songs about being one of the 'Tottenham boys making all the noise', or the 'Shoreham boys at Bramall Lane', because the songs don't include them.

Lifelong Tottenham fan and co-chair of Proud Lilywhites Chris Paouros tells me she physically bristles every time White Hart Lane launches into that chant. 'I don't sing it because it's predicated on you being a man,' she says, exasperated. 'It's like, well, we're not all boys, so think about that for a moment. I hardly go to away games now, because the levels of casual racism, sexism and homophobia are so horrendous. I'm quite mouthy so I usually say something, especially if it's a home game because I do feel that Tottenham is my home now – I've turned up without my season ticket before and still been let in because they know me there. But you can see it in people's eyes when they're thinking, "If I'd wanted a woman to moan at me I'd have stayed at home."'

Despite that, Chris and every other female fan I know still loves football. They endure the challenges, and keep going to the games. Why? Supporting Tottenham has been a constant in Chris's family life for over forty years. 'My granny couldn't read or write when she came to North London from Cyprus, but she taught herself to recognize the word "Tottenham" on the telly so she could understand the football scores and know if her son would come home happy or not.' Football became ingrained in her family – FA Cup days were a tradition, with 'posh' smoked salmon bridge rolls served in the front room so three generations could all sit around the TV. Football meant becoming part of British culture, making North London a home for future generations. That is no small detail. As an adult, White Hart Lane has become home to Chris. She has sat next to the same people for years. 'I know their routines intimately. At forty-two minutes one of them always gets up and says, "Do you want lager or bitter, John?" And the other says, "I don't know, Danny, what you having?" For fifteen years my wife, Monica, and I went to football together, and sat alongside these guys. I never saw them outside of football. But when Mon died, every single one of them came to her funeral.'

Chris ruminates on the inherent contradictions of our national game, how it can be a home, a constant – even though stadiums, players, kit, managers all change. And how it can be a comforting place, despite some of the worst forms of abuse. For a lesbian, in particular, men's football isn't an obvious place to find a home – all the homophobic abuse, for one thing – but Chris thinks it's something to do with having an identity. 'We joke about things being a bit "Spurs-y", that element of bonkers pride in finishing fourth and still not getting into the Champions League – who the fuck else does that? That's Spurs-y.'

Chris is determined to lead on the change she wants to see. As a lesbian who enjoys watching men's football, she was not only fed up with the bigotry she heard in the stands, but tired of football's LGBT groups that sought to represent only men's views. She felt it was time to ensure that lesbians had a stake in the conversation too. In her work for Proud Lilywhites, and the sport's umbrella group Pride in Football, Chris has been keen to ensure that tackling homophobia in football is not an exclusively male preserve. There are co-chairs, for gender parity, and an emphasis on reaching out to women to increase their involvement in the organization. She says she hopes her work will help to enable footballers to come out, if they wish. And she vents her frustration that even in the women's game there is not enough openness around sexuality. In the late 1990s Chris ran the legendary Hackney Women's FC, the first out lesbian team. Things have changed massively in the LGBT movement since then, but still there is a shyness in being open about sexuality – even in women's football. Coming out was a major event for England star Casey Stoney, and Chris wishes more female players would feel comfortable enough to talk about these issues. She herself grew up in a Greek Cypriot family where her mum wasn't keen on her tomboy status, and even less so when Chris came out. Chris says it would have helped enormously to have England players to look up to who were open about their sexual orientation. 'It's a real shame that it's still not talked about. It needs to be normalized. I don't mean outing people, but highlighting the importance of inclusion.'

I find Chris's story inspiring because she is living proof of why we don't need to turn our backs on the sports we love, just because they might retain archaic and unpleasant elements. There are plenty of people – men and women – who want sport to be truly inclusive, truly family-friendly. These are individuals, like Chris, who feel passionately about implementing change, and instead of sitting around wondering whether it's ever going to happen, they just go off and do it themselves. This is precisely what we need more of in sport. We need more women to reclaim sport, on their own terms, to mould it into the image they want to see, to become the architects of a new sporting culture that is more generous, more compassionate, and no less fun.

It is a mantra that Judy Murray has followed her entire sporting career, whether that was struggling to play tennis in 1970s Scotland with the nation's paucity of facilities and expertise, or fighting to take her now-famous sons to the very top of the sport. She has always created her own paths, relied on her own resourcefulness, dug deep and got on with the job. She has had to: even after Andy won the junior US Open she still couldn't get Sport Scotland to fund him.

Along the way she has faced the opprobrium of the mainstream media who, for many years, insisted on depicting her as the omnipresent, but essentially clueless, 'pushy parent'. The caricature of the female supporting act is one that is habitually lumped onto all women associated with a sports star as wives, girlfriends or mothers. It is grossly sexist, and unfair. Most of the so-called WAGs that I have met are smart, articulate, educated and career-focused. Unlike the stereotype, very few see their marriage as their vocation. And yet as soon as they display a little chutzpah, show a little business sense, they're characterized as hard-nosed bitches controlling their husbands' lives. Two high-profile examples are Mirka Federer and Tania Farah, wives of Roger Federer and Mo Farah, respectively. Two talented women juggling family and managing their husbands' careers, they are both frequently portrayed as some kind of modern-day Lady Macbeth. Fabrice Muamba's wife, Shauna, is another important female figure – running her own Caribbean sauce business, Mrs Muamba's, and holding the family together while her husband recovers from the moment when his heart stopped for seventy-eight minutes on the pitch at White Hart Lane, and a nation held its breath. Fabrice made a miraculous recovery, but it was Shauna who had to step into the role of breadwinner as her husband adjusted to a life without football.

Mums of sports stars don't necessarily have it any easier. From Cissie Charlton, mother of 1966 World Cup winning sons Jack and Bobby, to Sandra St Helen, mum of Jermain Defoe, mothers in sport tend to be portrayed as overbearing and interfering. When Jermain moved to Canada to play for Toronto FC in the MLS, a *Toronto Sun* journalist dedicated an entire column to the subject of his 'tantrum'-prone mum, cast as the wrecking ball in Defoe's professional career. It's just not the same for dads. Think of Bert le Clos, the father of Chad, who beat Michael Phelps to a gold medal in the pool at London 2012. From the sidelines, Bert went ballistic and became an instant media hit. He ended up becoming more famous than his medal-winning son, and the public adored him.

Judy, meanwhile, has had a very different path. 'I got

slammed a lot along the way for being "the mum" and being told I'm pushy and all the rest of it,' she told me. 'I just had to remind myself that the people who wrote these things don't know us, they've never spoken to me or my family; all they see is me pumping my fist in the box and they clearly think I'm some sort of crazy, psychotic mother and it couldn't be further from the truth.' The reality is that Judy has had to graft every step of the way, both in her own tennis career and in coaching her sons to play tennis through the early years. Scotland was never a hub of tennis talent; there was a lack of people to go to for advice, a lack of financial support, a lack of facilities and resources, and a lack of belief that anyone Scottish could ever become world class. Frustrated, she ended up quitting her job as national coach, and going it alone in developing her sons' skills. 'I did it by myself because I thought nobody will believe in my kids unless I do. It was a huge learning experience for me; I had to learn all sorts of things. I did a PR course so I didn't have to pay other people to do it, because I didn't have any money; I learned how to build a website; I can do tax returns in three different countries; I started to learn the life and the business to it. It's been a big adventure.' I say that most people don't know these things about her; they probably assume she did a bit of ball practice with the boys and then sat in the box at Wimbledon, hair done, cheering. 'Well, I never told anybody any of these things on the way up,' she says. 'I never did interviews, I just kept focused on what I was trying to do. It's only really in the last few years, with Andy winning slams, that I felt confident talking about it.'

As her words sink in, I can't help but feel she has been dealt an unfair hand. If a father had produced two sons as talented as

Andy and Jamie, and endured financial and emotional hardship to get them onto an elite platform, he would be hailed as a genius. Think of Lewis Hamilton's dad, frequently credited with the career of his son; the stories about him working several jobs to give Lewis a fighting chance in an elitist sport are well known. Why hasn't the same compliment been extended to Judy?

Like her son Andy, Judy is often portrayed in the media as rather dour. But a few minutes into our conversation and I realize she is anything but. A cake obsessive, she has me in stitches describing how she makes 'top hats' for her sons every time they come home. 'You couldn't really call it baking,' she says, 'but it's where you melt the chocolate, put it in the base of the cake case, split a marshmallow, put a blob of chocolate on top of it and a Smartie on top and it looks like a top hat. It's a real kids' party thing. At Andy's wedding I made thousands of them, but they were absolutely decimated between Jamie, Andy and Jamie Delgado. It brought back all their memories of children's parties. It was really funny; you're so used to seeing them in this elite sporting environment and there they were sitting round this tray of top hats talking about kids' party food.' We talk about lemon meringue pie, Victoria sponge and Coburg cake. It is one of Judy's favourite subjects, and I delight in chatting about cake as opposed to nutrition and protein shakes as is the norm with so many sports stars. Judy says these things are an important part of her family life. 'As a family we have very little time together; the boys don't get home much, so those moments are very precious. At Christmastime I always do party poppers and whoopee cushions and daft things like that; they make us laugh and reminisce.'

As her sons' success grew, Judy began to be approached by women's sports organizations asking her to help them fight gender inequality in their sector. As Fed Cup captain, Judy had begun to witness some of these issues herself. 'I realized how much harder it is to work and push to make things happen on the women's side of the game than the men's. Everything is very much focused on the men. Everybody talks about the Davis Cup; it has a bigger profile, it's been around longer, and in more prominent locations. There's hardly any female coaches on the women's tour, and of course hardly any on the men's – although Andy taking on Amélie [Mauresmo] has helped enormously in challenging those perceptions that women should be considered.'

Still, standing up and speaking at conferences, or to the media, wasn't something that felt comfortable. When Women in Sport announced that just 0.4 per cent of sponsorship went into women's sport, Judy was horrified. 'But at the time I said, oh God, no, I couldn't talk about anything that's not tennis. I said there must be someone else who can, I'm not confident in front of cameras. Isn't there another high-profile female coach, because I didn't think of myself in that way. And they said to me, "Well, can you think of anyone?" And I couldn't.' Judy agreed to sit down with the research, and the more she read the more angry she became. 'Angry and disappointed,' she says now. 'I knew women were well in the minority but I didn't realize how bad it was.' With no women on the board of the International Tennis Federation, women making up less than 1 per cent of FIFA's voting congress, and only one woman on the board of the Football Association, there is still a long way to go before women are even sitting at the table, let alone equally represented.

The stark figures prompted Judy into action. If no one else would speak up, she reasoned, then she simply had to. 'And so I've since made myself do things like that, because I've realized I do have a voice; I think it is important to have women in key positions so that [other] women can see it's possible. It's still not really my thing, I'm not gagging to get up and do it, it makes me very edgy, but I've become more confident in recent years. I felt more comfortable talking about how we'd come from a tiny town in Scotland and gone on this great big adventure and come out on the top of it. There were things on that journey that made it difficult for me because I was female, because I was their mum. Some things bothered me, but I never let anybody see that it did. I kept going because I wasn't going to get distracted by all that.'

I love that Judy grabbed the bull by the horns and decided to be part of the change she wanted to see. As a high-profile person she could easily have dodged the responsibility. But she felt passionately enough to want to make a difference. I felt that the first time I met her in person, at the launch of the Women's Sport Trust, where she spoke from the floor, railing against the lack of female coaches across sport and the injustices therein. I was genuinely taken aback by her commitment to the issues, and inspired. Best of all, she is not just a woman of words, but a woman of action.

In 2014, spurred on by frustrating experiences at the elite end of women's tennis, Judy decided to launch Miss Hits, a programme aimed at encouraging girls to play tennis, and women to coach. With four times as many boys coming into the sport as girls, Judy knew that women's elite tennis in Britain would never change until something was done about the grass-roots game. Most people would wait for a governing body to sort out a programme for them, but Judy is a roll-your-sleeves-up-and-get-on-with-it sort of person. 'I just felt that if I went and spoke to the LTA it would take forever to get off the ground,' she says, frankly. 'Like everything I've done and had success with, I've just done it myself.'

Judy invested £300K of her own money into starting up the scheme, which broke tennis down into a game with no rules. 'Tennis is a very complex coordination sport and you have little girls coming along for the first time who have never even held a racket in their hands – they don't know how to hold it, it's probably too heavy for them. We have to teach the skills first, how to throw and catch a bouncing ball, how to move to and from a bouncing ball, before thinking about hitting it. From the research we did it became clear that girls didn't like the way that boys were too competitive and too noisy and hit the ball too hard.'

The concept of breaking a sport down into bite-sized pieces that assumes no prior knowledge is so important. When it came to sport at school I always felt I had missed a trick somewhere. The boys all seemed to know what to do; I was already behind the curve even at primary school age. In my view, this is one of the greatest barriers to getting young girls interested in sport – that they are thrown in head first, and expected to muddle along. No wonder so few excel or enjoy it. Judy's approach echoes the same emphasis on physical literacy that Tanni talks about, or that Jacqui takes her young daughter to learn about at play schemes – creating the building blocks for the future. I count the months until my own daughter turns five and can join Judy's scheme. I think she'd love it. Already Miss Hits has trained up 200 teachers, which Judy says is a key part of the programme. 'Female coaches love the fact that it's just for girls, and just for them. So often in tennis we're outnumbered as female coaches; women are squeezed out or shut up. They're in a minority so they don't have the confidence to speak up or ask questions.'

Judy knows first hand how important it is to have faith in female coaches, and it is a belief she appears to have instilled in her sons too. When Andy appointed Amélie Mauresmo as his coach it made global headlines, so rare was it to see a female coach working at the highest level in men's sport – never mind that Amélie had won Wimbledon and the Australian Open in her own playing career. As he struggled to make a comeback from injury, the results didn't go his way at first, and he gallantly made a point of defending his coach from the barbed criticism aimed in her direction. He saw it for what it was: thinly veiled prejudice, and bravely decided that he was having none of it.

In 2015 Andy took the extraordinary step of writing a comment piece for *L'Équipe* defending his appointment of Amélie. 'Have I become a feminist?' he wrote. 'Well, if being a feminist is about fighting so that a woman is treated like a man then yes, I suppose I have.' It was an incredible moment, the very embodiment of #HeForShe as a reality and not just a social media hashtag. Andy instantly earned the respect of many more female fans and commentators. That same year, in the US, there were more female firsts in men's sport – the San Antonio Spurs hired Becky Hammon, making her the NBA's first-ever full-time female coach in history, swiftly followed by the Sacramento

King's appointment of Nancy Lieberman, making her only the second part-time female coach in the history of the sport; in the NFL Jen Welter became the sport's first female hire for the Arizona Cardinals; meanwhile Sarah Thomas became the first full-time female NFL referee. But Andy and Amélie's story was something special, a personal relationship in which he spoke up for her against the critics, and didn't bat an eyelid when she went on maternity leave. 'With Amélie it was a brave choice in some ways,' says Judy. 'It is very unusual to find female coaches working with anyone at that level in men's sport, but in other ways it was a no-brainer because she has a similar outlook and feel for the game. She's been at the top, she knows the emotions, she knows how hard you have to work, and she hasn't got an ego. She sits and she listens to Andy and lets him talk, and I think at this stage of his life that was one of the things he was looking for, to be more open about how he felt about everything.'

And therein lies the reason why it is so very short-sighted to deny women opportunities in sport. Because women contribute something that's unique. And while it might be more comfortable to persist with the old ways, to wriggle out of challenging sexism, to resist building extra female toilets in sports stadiums, it isn't more productive. It isn't what's best for sport. I go to a lot of women and sport forums, and read a lot about why gender inequality exists. And one of the most common things I hear is that women aren't confident enough. They don't put themselves forward for things, they don't apply for jobs, they don't ask for pay rises, they don't insist on promotions. There is truth in this, for sure. But it's also the lazy verdict. It plays into our image of women as weak, lacking in leadership and the skills needed for success. And why would you want to employ anyone who hasn't got what it takes to overcome these issues?

I was fascinated to read a different slant on this whole debate in the *Harvard Business Review*. Society's idea of success, it argued, was based on male attributes. What society didn't recognize was where these attributes frequently let us down, when male leaders were overly aggressive, too comfortable with risk-taking, confident without basis. Why, it asked, did we not value the qualities that women bring to the table? Why did we eternally see elements, such as Amélie's ability to listen to Andy, as a weakness?

I find it exciting to see the change taking place in sport right now, in our lifetimes. Sure, at times it is frustratingly slow. I get annoyed when sport institutionally, habitually, sidelines women and minorities. But I am cheered by all the individual exceptions to this trend. By the Judys, the Andys, the Amélies, the Annies and the Chrises who are taking decisions into their own hands and shaping sport into a world they want to be part of. They are, collectively, making things better. Not just because it is morally the right thing to do, but because it is part of evolution, innovation, progress, and pushing sport to new heights. They are making sport better. We must congratulate their efforts, and – ultimately – join them.

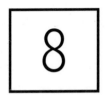

8

What does a woman's voice in sport sound like?
(And when can we stop pretending to be blokes?)

I first realized that football existed in my primary school play-ground, aged six, watching an enormous group of boys kick a ball about on the concrete. I clocked the game, and promptly went back to pretending to be a squirrel. On a bicycle. Playing football, I decided there and then, was clearly something that boys did, and girls didn't do. How they ever learned this game was invisible to me. Football, I thought, must just be an innate skill that boys possessed. So I carried on with the squirrel game, and didn't think any more of it.

Forever after, football was a game that I missed out on learn-ing how to play. Because football, I figured, well, any sport really, was either something imbued in you, or it wasn't. So when I was twelve and secondary school introduced a term of football into our PE lessons, I had already decided that it was too late to learn. And when a bunch of girls started playing at university, I thought it was *definitely* too late to learn. And when some of my friends started playing in our late twenties, I was adamant that there was just no point. At every stage in my life, football and I had missed the boat.

Perhaps it could never have been otherwise. When I was growing up on a street in Camden Town, North London, there wasn't any sport going on. The park at the end of the road was taken over by traveller caravans each summer, and the local kids preferred knock down ginger to knocking a ball about. The only live action was the Stag's Head pub over the road – fights, arguments, smashing, yelling. On hot summer nights, my bedroom window open to let in the cool night air, I'd lie in bed listening to the drink-infused dramas. The next morning there would be broken glass outside our house and my mum would be out, cursing, with a brush and pan to clean it up.

In our own house sport was near enough a dirty word. My dad had grown up in sports-mad South Africa, following the exploits of Manchester United and the test cricket on the radio, but his interest in football died a death the day he went to his first football match in England in 1976. Having just quit his home country in protest at the racial segregation laws and violence under apartheid, he was horrified to discover that English football was a hotbed of hooliganism. He visited Filbert Street and, on approach to the stadium, saw shops and houses boarded up, bracing themselves for trouble. He swore never to return to a football stadium. Meanwhile South Africa was banned from playing international sport, and it would be almost another two decades before my dad could comfortably celebrate his home country hosting, and winning, the 1995 rugby World Cup.

In many ways the requirements for being a sports fan are as embryonic as playing sport itself. If you don't have a team to support before you can walk, you're not seen as a true supporter.

It's as though if you're not there from the very start, from before you can even consciously grant consent to being a sports fan in the first place, then you can never truly be accorded the title of 'proper supporter'. It's kind of an in-utero-or-you're-out type conundrum.

The problem with this pedant's quest for authenticity of course, is that it's really just code for 'bloke'. Everything other is deemed wrong. And that, I surmise, is the reason for women sounding so weird at football matches. Myself included. As the crowd stirs to a chant, instinctively a sound emerges from my throat that is as low as my voice can go; a faux drunken roar, and a slur. That's how I sound at football. Occasionally I have hit a few notes in my native vocal range, and promptly stuttered. A series of strange squeaks, like a boy adapting to manhood, voice officially broken. In the end, though, I can only feel comfortable at football singing like a man. And yet that is – by definition – intensely uncomfortable.

Maybe that's because there isn't a proper cultural space for women to be football fans. Take Nick Hornby's iconic football memoir *Fever Pitch*, for example, an intense and brilliantly written narrative about being an Arsenal fan. On its publication in 1992 everyone was raving about this incredible book, which was fast becoming a totemic symbol of the intellectualization and new middle-class acceptability of football. As an Arsenal fan I knew I was supposed to love it, but I didn't. How could I love a book where women were portrayed as nagging, irritating diversions from the football? Damn their reproductive organs! Must they insist on giving birth before full time? 'How was I supposed to get excited about the oppression of females if they couldn't be trusted to stay upright during the final minutes of a desperately close promotion campaign?' asks Nick Hornby's narrator.[29] Where was I, as a woman, supposed to fit into this apparently modern picture of football?

And that's why women stand out on match days, even in the twenty-first century. We're not written into the narrative, so when we do pop up – unexpectedly – everyone freaks and starts talking about kitchens. For this reason I feel a genuine sympathy for Delia Smith, celebrity cook and joint majority shareholder at Norwich City Football Club. The doyenne of cookery writing and one of Britain's national treasures, Delia, when she dared to raise her voice at a football match, was roundly ridiculed. Her now-infamous 2005 rallying cry at Norwich's home ground, Carrow Road, as the team drew level with Manchester City at half-time, was intended to be a display of passion. 'A message for the best football supporters in the world,' she yelled into the microphone, in exactly the kind of woman's football voice I am talking about, 'we need a twelfth man here. Where are you? Where are you? Let's be 'avin' you! Come on!' The next day the *Sun* newspaper accused her of being drunk, the *Independent* said she was a fool, and the *Mirror* thought she should be up for FA charges of bringing the game into disrepute. Meanwhile a section of the less charming Chelsea fans reportedly sang, 'We've got [Roman] Abramovich, you've got a drunken bitch.' No charges pressed.

Incredibly, to this day, Delia still finds her alcohol intake is monitored and commented on by journalists. Since when did shouting a bit at the football mean you're an alcoholic? Isn't that just what you're supposed to do? 'All my working career they called me a saint,' said Delia, reflecting on the hypocrisy, 'suddenly now I can only speak under the influence of alcohol

– absolute nonsense.' Was Delia drunk? Who knows. Maybe she was just a bit tipsy and shouting in a woman's version of a man's voice at the football. The truth is, it could have been any of us. As Delia put it at the time, 'I was just really, really caught up in what was happening with the football.' [30]

That's the thing about women at football: they are notice-able. Any mention of Arsenal's Highbury Screamer – a female fan famous for letting out an agonized scream when the team concede a goal – is met with vitriol on Internet fans' forums for her high-pitched efforts. In a blogger's list of 'Ten Things That Spoil The Beautiful Game', which included cheating and swear-ing at the referee, the Highbury Screamer was placed seventh – worse than hooliganism. 'Every time the players were near the net an almighty wail would rip through the crowd and split your eardrums,' opined the blogger. A brief trawl of fans' forums provides ample evidence of such attitudes, with supporters com-plaining about their female peers being too 'squeaky' and 'needing a punch' and wishing they would stay home to sort the dinner out.

Don't just take my word for it, ask a bloke. Specifically, one that used to be a woman. The writer behind the popular LadyArse.com fan's blog recently began a gender reassignment process and is now known as Lee Hurley. His blog also under-went a sex change and became the 'Daily Cannon'. Lee told the *Daily Mirror* about the difference in the responses from football fans since changing his gender. His experience is fascinating. 'When people disagree with my opinions they disagree with *me* now, not an entire gender. When I was writing as female I was called a "slut" and a "virgin" who "needs a good seeing to". "Wench", "whore", "lesbo" and "dyke" were all quite common insults . . . Writing as male, the insults have become more generic. I'm an "idiot", "moron", "asshole", all things I was also called when writing as female but without the "stupid f***ing female" prefix which was almost expected, I received it that often . . . With two different people, one male and one female, it is easy to dismiss the difference in abuse for a myriad factors. But when it is the *same person* and the nature of the abuse changes so radically, what else can it demonstrate?'[31]

The year I turned ten our lives changed forever. Though I'd grown up hating Margaret Thatcher, our family soon had her to thank as we benefited from the Conservative government's Right To Buy ruling and bought and sold the council flat we'd lived in for almost a decade. Instantly my family became upwardly mobile, residents of a more leafy way of life in North London's Crouch End. Or 'yuppies', as my brother scathingly put it. My mum and dad breathed a heavy sigh of relief – no more drug dens, police raids, prostitutes, domestic violence, scarred wrists, shouting, cider breath, L-O-V-E / H-A-T-E tattoos on knuckles, or walls so paper thin we could hear the neighbours' telly or even smell their dinner. Despite all the social horrors, though, my brother and I missed Camden Town desperately. As far as we were concerned it was real life, and our home. Bus-dependent Crouch End seemed a million miles away from anywhere.

But with the new North London territory came new sights and sounds too – the most striking of which was the proximity to Arsenal's old Highbury stadium. Soon after moving in I remember playing in my bedroom one sunny Saturday afternoon and hearing a roar. A thrilling chorus of human voices, crescendoing on the air. The air vibrated with the noise. 'What's that?' I asked my dad. 'Oh, Arsenal must have scored,' he said casually. I loved it.

'Football was just part of where we lived,' remembers one of my oldest schoolfriends, Clare, who grew up a short walk away from the old Arsenal ground. 'It wasn't ever a matter of, "it's for boys," it was all around us; you could hear the football lying in your bed, everyone at school talked about it, it was part of our community.' I love that Clare says this because, if you met her, you wouldn't think she was at all interested in sport. She doesn't talk about sport, doesn't watch sport, and doesn't play any sport. She hated PE at school where, because she was tall, they always tried to get her to do the high jump.

Twenty-five years on, though, she still remembers every word of 'Back Where We Belong', the 1989 title-winning Arsenal song with Paul Davis, Tony Adams and Lee Dixon singing their hearts out in high-waisted chinos. '*We're back!*' sings Clare now, picking at a quesadilla in trendy eaterie Wahaca, '*back where we bel-o-ng / We only had a minute but then we went and did it . . .* Doesn't everyone know that one? It's up there with the John Barnes rap, I thought . . . ?'

No doubt my secondary school had a big part to play in our football interest. It was a girls' school where we called our teachers 'Ms', and learned about suffragettes and Femidoms. Each tutor group was named after a different inspirational woman in history – from the world's first computer programmer, Ada Lovelace, to nineteenth-century social activist Annie Besant and Olympic gold medallist Tessa Sanderson. And while we didn't really play football, we were certainly obsessed with following it. The morning after Arsenal won the FA Cup in

1993 our school went Arsenal crazy. Scarves, shirts and flags hung out of the windows. No one got any work done that day, as a thousand girls erupted in uncontrollable excitement. It was a lovely feeling, being part of that achievement, all together.

The Arsenal obsession of my peers was best embodied by my friend Lucy. If it had Arsenal on it, she owned it. Arsenal scrunchies, Arsenal pencil cases, scarves, tops, badges and stickers: she was covered in them. She was a Neil Heaney fan. Never mind that he only ever played nine first-team games; as Lucy says, 'He was handsome. I waited around for his autograph on my wallet, and then covered it in sticky-back plastic.'

For Lucy, paradoxically, football has often felt like one of the safest spaces to be a woman. 'One of the most refreshing things for me about going to football as a girl is that the guys aren't looking at you,' she says now. 'They're looking at the football. It's one of the few places you can go as a woman and be at ease. When you go outside and you're in the crowd it starts again, of course; you get a few eyes or "phwoar"s, but not as much as you would anywhere else. I love that about football. Just not to get hassled by guys for ninety minutes while you're surrounded by them is really refreshing.' I know what she means. While the match is on there's often a hiatus where it feels as though no one notices the fact that you are a woman, all eyes focused on the pitch. You can meld into one crowd, rooting for the same outcome, united. It's not always that way, of course, but when it happens, it's an extraordinary feeling. You are a human being, identified only by your football colours, not your sex. It's a rare experience for women to have.

For a girl, knowing about football earned you respect from boys, and that brought confidence. Having boys eat out of your hand, bowing to your superior knowledge about sport, is pretty cool as a teenager. 'I remember one time watching an FA Cup game, and Arsenal were playing a team in another division,' Lucy says. 'Because it was a lower-league side they didn't have the names of the players on the back of their shirts. I remember my boyfriend at the time went, "That team's so poor they can't even afford to put names on the back of their shirts!" That was typical of him. Dissing everything in sight. And I said, "Um, isn't it because they're not Premier League?" I remember all the boys looked at each other and they were like, "Yeah, she's right, you know." And then they all started laughing and went, "Oh no! You just got told!"' She grins.

Lucy enjoyed knowing the answer to the football trivia that day. Who doesn't? But that pressure to know everything about sport puts a lot of women off defining themselves as sports fans. It's that idea that you can't just *like sport*, you've got to prove yourself as a proper fan. Your loyalty, authenticity, knowledge, are all up for scrutiny if you want to be accepted. It's a doctrine that affects men as well as women, of course, but women – as the perceived exceptions – are usually treated with a greater degree of suspicion and a more intense line of questioning. At times it can feel intimidating. Why would any sane person subject themselves to such a level of scrutiny just because they might fancy watching a bit of sport on the telly once in a while? No wonder so many women feel excluded.

But here's the thing: enjoying sport shouldn't be akin to joining a private members' club where you need to be vouched for, learn a secret knock, and possess a pair of testicles. Sport is meant to be fun. For everyone. The stats about goals scored, shutouts and strike rates don't really matter. Not knowing about them doesn't make you any less of a fan if your heart still pounds remembering the drama of Barnsley knocking Liverpool out of the FA Cup, but you just can't quite recall the scoreline. Maybe to some people that stuff matters. But sport is not only about statistics; it is just as much about drama, characters, unfolding plots, intrigue, transgression, heroics, passion, determination, luck, and those special moments of incredible jaw-dropping displays of human ability. You don't need to be born with a football yearbook in your mouth to appreciate these elements. And that's the message that I want to send to potential female sports fans, and the organizations that attempt to woo them. Women and girls are not dependent on baby-pink replica shirts, or club insignia oven gloves, or cocktails at the match; they are just as capable of enjoying the action with a Bovril and a bulky coat on. They just need to be made to feel welcome. And they need to be allowed to enjoy sport on their own terms, in their own way. Free from judgement.

A key part of the solution is making sure that women can physically access sport, whether that means architects including enough women's toilets in sports stadia, or accommodating parents' needs with a crèche – as Chelsea do at Stamford Bridge – or making provision for babies to be allowed in the stands. Ahead of the recent rugby World Cup in England I was thrilled to hear from so many mums and dads desperate to bring their babies with them to the matches. They contacted me because they were devastated to discover that babes in arms were not allowed into World Cup stadia unless they had a ticket – even though many of the babies hadn't even been conceived when their parents originally bought tickets for the tournament. They rang customer services in their droves, only to be told either that all the tickets for their matches had sold out, or that they would have to pay over £200 – for a baby to attend! I thought this was insane, and – as several parents pointed out – discriminatory, particularly to breastfeeding mothers. Some of the parents were travelling from as far afield as New Zealand, Australia, the USA, Germany and France. Initially there was apathy towards this situation from the authorities. One very senior woman in sport told me, 'Well, the mums will just have to stay home.' I was horrified. Not only did this seem grossly unfair and lacking in equality, but on reading all these personal emails from parents I was getting such a lovely picture of families enjoying watching sport together. They told me how many years they'd all been attending games, how husband and wife always sat together, and as each child joined the family so they came along too. One mum said she'd be happy to leave her baby with the grandma, but she was already volunteering in the fans' zone. Clearly, the whole family was rugby crazy. How could we be letting down such dedicated fans? It seemed to go against everything we had been trying to achieve in encouraging women and families to attend sport.

Luckily I knew the brilliant Joanna Manning-Cooper, head of marketing at the World Cup, and she helped put me in touch with the head of ticketing. I probably drove the poor man insane forwarding all these desperate pleas from rugby fans with breastfed babies, just a few days away from the start of the biggest tournament in the sport. But all credit to him: he promised me that they would ensure that no one missed out, promptly making alternative arrangements so that all parents with babes in arms could collect a free ticket on the day of the match for their little ones to attend. The resolution made so many fans happy, families who were eager to share this special sporting moment with those closest to them, but I can't help but wonder why such considerations aren't an essential part of every sporting experience. I remember going to London 2012 with my then ten-month-old daughter, and grinning from ear to ear when I stumbled upon a buggy park. Not only was it a brilliant practical solution in accommodating families with young children and their bulky prams, but it sent such a clear message to sports fans: you are all welcome here; the fact that you are a parent is not an inconvenience.

I wish the same could be said for disabled supporters. A campaign to enable disabled sports fans to access stadia has been valiantly fought by Women in Football board member Joyce Cook for over a decade now. In 2014, seventeen Premier League clubs out of twenty did not provide an adequate number of spaces for wheelchairs, and there were reports of supporters having walking sticks and aids taken away from them on entering some grounds, and of families being separated into disabled and non-disabled areas. Can you imagine taking your disabled child to the football and being told you will not be able to sit together? Thankfully, Joyce, chair of Level Playing Field, went public with her frustrations and the Equality and Human Rights Commission took up the cause; meanwhile the issues were raised in parliament. The Premier League have now promised to comply with the Accessible Stadia Guide by 2017.

In spite of all the nonsense, women have been carving out their own space as fans for decades – from Rihanna tweeting about the World Cup, to Keira Knightley being interviewed about former Manchester United defender Gary Neville's Sky Sports punditry. 'He is just fucking amazing! Absolutely fucking

amazing!' says Keira, a West Ham fan who watches football on
her laptop when she's in Hollywood, and bought a TV especially so that she could watch games back in the UK. Then
there's Queen of Cakes Mary Berry, a huge Bath Rugby fan
who likes to spend a Saturday afternoon down at the Rec, and
Lily Allen who loves test cricket, and J. K. Rowling who seems
to tweet about every sport going, from tennis at Wimbledon to
the rugby World Cup. I wish we heard more about all these
sport-loving celebrities. There's endless pages of coverage about
them on the red carpet, with glamorous outfits, or intense analysis of their fashion choices or their love lives, but hardly a
word written about their interest in sport. Why not? How
refreshing it would be to see a full-length interview with J. K.
Rowling about sport on TV, or hear Mary Berry talk about
wrapping up warm for games at the Rec, instead of speculative
commentary on who she's flirted with most on the *Bake Off*. If
young girls could see the biggest female stars talking excitedly
about sport it would have a huge knock-on effect on their own
interest. It would recast glamorous celebrities as central to the
sporting action, not simply gorgeous sidekicks to a potential
sporting romance. Imagine if Keira was invited onto a sports
quiz show, or interviewed as part of the coverage? Clare Balding
does this to great effect in her horse racing coverage for Channel 4, where she walks around the racecourse bumping into
celebrities and chatting with them about their race tips. I'd love
to see more of that happening in mainstream sport.

Bestselling crime writer Val McDermid would make a great
interviewee. Her father was a scout for Raith Rovers and
discovered the legendary midfielder Jim Baxter, one of Scotland's greatest-ever players. Val spent her formative years on

the sidelines of muddy football pitches with her dad, watching miners and shipyard workers kicking lumps out of each other. 'He used to take me with him to get me out from under my mum's feet,' she told me, laughing. 'My dad would carry a plank of wood in the car so that in the wintertime we wouldn't sink ankle-deep in the mud. We went to Stark's Park occasionally too. The first memory I have is sitting on a railing, freezing cold in the winter, and then getting a hot pie and the gravy running down the inside of my sleeve, and thinking, "Ooh, that's lovely."' Val chuckles. 'They still do a good pie at Rovers. It's a crucial part of football.' I'm lost as she starts on about pies with macaroni cheese or baked beans. 'Have you never had a bean and potato pie?' she asks, incredulous. 'You've not lived!'

Val liked watching the football, but more often than not she would end up entertaining herself – a fiction writer in the making. 'When I was a kid being bored was a part of childhood, really. There was no expectation that children would be entertained every minute of the day. From a very early age I learned the exercise of imagination. I'd make up stories and amuse myself that way.'

When Val's dad passed away aged sixty-four, Val was just thirty-two. The loss was immense, but there was one place in the world where Jim McDermid lived on, and that was Raith Rovers. Like *Sex and the City* actress Kim Cattrall, whose father was a passionate Liverpool supporter, forging a surprising but intimate connection between the Hollywood star and Anfield, Val was drawn closer to her dad through the club. And I don't mean that in a sentimental way. Jim literally lives on through the club because Rovers fans won't forget him. Every time they see Val they remind her of just how important her dad was to them.

'As far as Kirkaldy is concerned, it doesn't matter how many books I sell or how many prizes I win, I'll always just be Jim McDermid's lassie. There's a very fine fish and chip shop in Kirkaldy called Valenti's. I went in the other day and John Valenti was frying; he called over one of his staff and he said, "You support the Rovers don't you?" and the woman said yes. And he said, "Well, this woman's father discovered Jim Baxter!" Not: this woman's an international bestselling lesbian cultural icon or anything like that,' she laughs riotously. 'Oh no, no. And so I'm very aware of coming back to a place where I was. There's a saying in Scotland: "I kent her faither," which means, "I knew her father." It's about keeping people connected to where they belong. For me it's been very much a retying to my roots, I suppose.'

That reconnecting manifested itself in a literal way when Gordon Brown, a fellow Rovers fan, contacted Val to help drum up some sponsorship for the club. She ended up financing one of the stands . . . and the home kit. It must be the first professional football kit in history to have a woman's name emblazoned across the front: ValMcDermid.com. The news went everywhere, and Val still sounds stunned that shirt sponsorship of a club in the Scottish Championship would receive worldwide attention. 'I was on TV, in the newspapers, on the radio, I even had the *New York Times* on the phone asking about it. And I've really noticed the number of times I've been stopped in the street by middle-aged men since then, and they say, "I'm not a fan of your club but I think what you're doing is great and I've started reading your books, by the way . . . !" so it works. It's a win–win.' But the link is more than a financial one. 'It gives me a different place, a place where I'm judged by different criteria. I like the fact it gives me another world to be in. As a writer you're always looking for material and that comes from a lot of places, and it does open that door to another world, a world I wouldn't normally come into contact with in my life.'

It can be hard to explain quite what's so special or meaningful about sport, but Val articulates it beautifully as she talks about why football takes such a central position in so many people's lives. 'I suppose if you can watch football and remain optimistic there's a fair chance you can get through life and remain optimistic,' she laughs. 'Life is tough, and full of disappointments for people. Having a team that you can pin some hope on, and every Saturday at the home games you sit with the same bunch of people who share that optimism – and those moments of grief and despair – with you, there's a real solidarity among the hardcore fans who come every week. We all need a place in our lives where we feel supported and where we feel a sense of solidarity.'

I ask Val if, as a lesbian and a rare example of a woman in the director's box, she ever encounters hostility or a sense of not belonging in football. 'I think because I walked through the door with a cheque in my hand they were very pleased to have me,' she laughs. 'The general view of our supporters can be summed up by saying, "You might be a lesbian, but you're *our* lesbian." No one's ever said that, but that's how it seems to me. A little while ago – it still cracks me up – I was at a home game and walking back to the south stand with the home end chanting, "You fat bastard!" at someone on the pitch. As I walked past, one of the guys caught my eye and he went, "It's not you we're talking about, Val." I thought that was great!

'I've actually never had homophobic abuse or any problem in the game. I have had occasions where I've been in the board-room and another director has come in and spoken to the male director on my left and the male director on my right and his eyes have just slid over me as if I don't exist, but I think that's just to do with me being a woman and not anything else.' She seems chuffed to bits that the fans find her approachable, and that she is in a position to make changes for them, even small ones. She roars with laughter at the memory of a woman who stopped her in the airport one day. 'She said, "You're Val McDermid, aren't you? I go to the Rovers every Saturday I can manage, and can I tell you it's a real disgrace there's never any soap in the ladies' toilets." Well, I took this to the board and I said, "It's a disgrace there's no soap in the ladies' toilets – some-thing of which I was unaware." And now we do have soap in the ladies' toilets.' Val beams. 'These are wee things but they make a difference to people.' Val hits the nail on the head. Soap in the ladies toilets *does* make a difference. It sends out a mes-sage that the experience of their female fans is of as much importance as that of their male fans. I bet that same woman was delighted, the next time she visited Stark's Park, to find full soap dispensers in the ladies'.

Some of the best female football fans I have ever met are those who have gone to football for decades – from England World Cup glory in 1966, gritting their teeth through the hoo-ligan years, and out again the other side, oblivious to what anyone else thought about the presence of females. Often they are stalwarts of their club, like non-league Kettering Town fans

Anne and Molly, who run the club shop (proudly selling £3 'I scored at Rockingham Road' knickers). 'We're like Hinge and Bracket, Anne and I,' Molly told me, 'the French and Saunders of non-league football.'[32] Anne and Molly have been going to football since they were 'old enough to look over the wall', watching with fascination as Paul Gascoigne took over as manager for a media-frenzied thirty-nine-day spell. I enjoy their cheeky confidence, mocking their husbands' timid affiliations with the Poppies. 'My husband is a fan but I don't let him come to matches,' Anne told me. 'When he does they lose dramatically, so he's banned. He doesn't mind being banned as long as he can watch the telly, because it's usually cold anyway. They're fair-weather supporters, aren't they? We go all weathers, we do.' I love how much fun the pair seem to have together, giggling their way through our interview, remembering the good times and the bad, with football a central part of their friendship that spans so many years. Then there's the inimitable Esme Stokes, now in her eighties, who was married at half-time on her local football pitch, given a Sky Sports subscription for her sixtieth wedding anniversary, and does the teas and squash for the club: 'I hammer on the door and say I'm coming in whether you're in the shower or not.' The very existence of these women challenges the notion that female fans in football – in sport – are a modern phenomenon. They are not. I only wish we made more of them, gave them a platform to become fan role models for younger generations of women and girls who might otherwise be put off.

I'd certainly love to know their view on a woman's voice at the match. Or on the telly, in view of the furore when Jacqui Oatley became the first woman to commentate on English football's iconic highlights programme, *Match of the Day*, in 2007. We probably should have seen it coming, after the Delia stuff, but I honestly didn't. When I speak to Jacqui now, we laugh at our naivety. I'll never forget her calling me up on a sunny spring day to tell me she'd been offered a TV game to commentate on, and me whooping like crazy on the other end of the phone. For her, the sexism angle was never more than a flicker of a thought, she recalls. 'I do remember saying in passing to the *Match of the Day* editor ahead of my first game, "I wonder whether it will be picked up on . . ."' We laugh riotously. 'It sounds silly now, but I didn't really think of it as being that big a deal from a gender perspective.'

One of the hardest facts for her to swallow, even now, is that so few people gave her credit for all the hard work she had put in to get the role, working her way up from hospital radio to a postgraduate degree in journalism and covering the non-league scene, standing at windy grounds without press boxes, doing commentary down a mobile phone. And then all the experience she gained at BBC 5 Live doing national commentary on the radio. One of the most hard-working, professional and con-scientious people I have ever met in football, Jacqui takes football prep to anorak levels. I always looked forward to her radio commentaries, and her appointment made total sense to me. But a few days before her debut some joyless git decided to leak the information to the newspapers, and a national debate ensued.

'Everything was fine until the Tuesday before the Saturday of the game and this little article appeared in the *Daily Mail*, a tiny snippet about me being the first woman to do *Match of the Day*. I remember thinking, "Oh no, it's got out before the

Saturday," but even then I didn't think it would get blown up to such an extent. On a flight back from Italy I was sat next to [BBC 5 Live presenter] Eleanor Oldroyd. I remember discussing it with her and my heart sinking. I sat there staring straight ahead thinking, "Oh jeez, I hope this doesn't turn out to be a big deal."' The next day there was a full-page spread in the *Daily Mail* and a debate over whether women should be allowed to commentate on football matches. By Thursday it was front-page news in the *Telegraph*. 'The *Guardian* had a big photo and a headline saying, "Is football ready for Jacqui Oatley?" I was thinking it's 2007, wow. And anyway, what do you mean, is football ready? I've already been doing this job on radio for years.

'On the Wednesday morning I remember waking up to my radio alarm clock, which is always set to 5 Live, and it was my good friend Rachel Burden reading the headlines. The top-of-the-hour item included a debate on whether a woman should be allowed to commentate on *Match of the Day*. I remember lying in bed thinking, "Oh my gosh, my own radio station, who I work for, is actually running a news piece on whether I should be allowed to commentate on *Match of the Day*?" I couldn't believe it. I was absolutely astonished. I kept thinking: "But I work for you!" I was in the middle of this brewing storm and I felt very much on my own. It was a really strange feeling.'

Over the next few days Jacqui's phone didn't stop ringing. For a prep anorak, the constant interruptions were a nightmare. Plus there were all the other things to worry about. At one point, while she was on the phone to her mum in Wolverhampton, she heard a knock at the door. 'My mum said, "Hang on, darling, the doorbell's just gone," and I overheard her politely declining whoever it was, and she came back on the line and said, "Oh sorry, darling, that was just the *News of the World*, they wanted some photos of you playing football as a child . . ."' Meanwhile friends of Jacqui's received phone calls from journalists asking for information. One tabloid wanted to know, 'Is Jacqui a lesbian?'

The themes up for 'discussion' were prehistoric. Would a woman's voice be suitable for the job? Former Wimbledon FC manager Dave Bassett was concerned for the reputation of football. 'Maybe the BBC are trying to be innovative and groundbreaking, but I think it undermines the credibility of the programme and when she commentates at the weekend I will not be watching,' said Dave. 'I never really agreed that we should have women officials and I don't think we should have female commentators. And my wife agrees.'

Cameron Carter, writing for football magazine *When Saturday Comes*, described Jacqui's debut as akin to 'the earnest trilling of a schoolboy competition winner', before going on to say that 'her summary of the game was, as you might expect, entirely satisfactory.' He did note, however, the many complaints from online bloggers, including, 'The male ear is not tuned to comfortable reception of the treble clef.'[33] Which is a strange thing to say. Does the blogger mean that all female speech is uncomfortable for men to listen to? 'It seems this country contains thousands of middle-aged men who hide, barely, a nervous physiological reaction to the sound of the female voice,' Carter concluded. Damningly, even some of the women joined in – Julie Welch, herself a female pioneer as the first-ever female football reporter on a national newspaper, said that Jacqui could only be successful 'if she can make us forget she's female'.

Is that what women in football have to be, then? Women in disguise as men? I think that's a terrible indictment of our cultural attitudes towards women in male-dominated environments. When we look at fashion, no one says Ralph Lauren or Giorgio Armani should butt out of women's clothing design, we just appreciate their work. Shouldn't it be the same for women working in men's sport? Jacqui's addition to the *Match of the Day* line-up catapulted the show into the twenty-first century and promised so much for the future of match commentary, a craft often lambasted for being overly clichéd and stale. We swoon at the progress that Premier League football has made in the last twenty years – the speed of play, the skilfulness of the players, the overall fitness. Surely we want our match commentators to progress too?

One of the greatest innovations in modern football punditry has come through Gary Neville's match footage analysis on Sky Sports. The level of detail he brings to his descriptions provides a fascinating insight. It's a huge departure from the tired analysis we've had for years; Gary brings excitement, and a new way of doing things. One of my favourite TV moments of 2014 was watching him get out of his seat, pull up his suit trousers and pretend to be Liverpool goalkeeper Simon Mignolet, squatting close to the ground, acting out his hypothesis. As a reporter Jacqui has provided her own groundbreaking moments in football coverage. Her 2014 post-match interview with Arsène Wenger for *Match of the Day* is a great example of what she brings as a broadcaster. It was hailed as brilliant and courageous journalism, asking the probing questions that her colleagues rarely dare to ask of an established manager like Wenger, but unfortunately that didn't stop her from being subjected to a torrent of abuse on social media. While the likes of Gary Lineker and Piers Morgan defended her, others let rip. But they were missing the point. Sport and sports coverage thrives off innovation, and the more we embrace it the better quality entertainment we will have. Sadly, for too many people, the fact that Jacqui is female remained an insurmountable obstacle to them ever opening their ears and listening to what she actually had to say.

'It just really highlighted how much mistrust people had at the time of a woman being able to do that job, or having the passion, knowledge and experience,' says Jacqui now of her *Match of the Day* debut. 'Maybe if Twitter had been more popular at the time they would have known I tweet about football all day every day; maybe they just thought I'd been plucked from the office and plonked in the commentary box and told to shout, "Yakubu!" A lot of it is quite amusing, people's perceptions. You realize actually what a lot of people genuinely thought about women in football. Hopefully times have changed since.'

So, have they? No woman has since commentated on the BBC's flagship football programme, or even on BBC 5 Live's football coverage. Jacqui's history-making first-ever *MOTD* commentary is preserved in the National Football Museum in Manchester as just that – a piece of history. Jacqui says life has changed a lot for her personally. She feels much more respected by those in the industry – managers, players, journalists. 'Maybe I've gained that level of acceptance for being around for so long. [But] I think one of the reasons I've become accepted is because I moved into presenting rather than staying in commentating. I think that is still an issue. I think a lot of people, and not just men, by the way, don't want to hear a woman commentate. There's the acceptance – does she really know what she's talking about? Can I trust her to tell me who's playing well and who's not? And that's an innate part of prejudice. People want to know: have you played the game? Dave Bassett's quote about not having kicked a ball in my life made me laugh; I changed career because I had to give up playing, and I'm a qualified coach. He just made an assumption!'

Jacqui hopes that the next woman to commentate on *MOTD* will face less opprobrium, simply by virtue of being the second rather than the first. She wonders, though, if any woman will be prepared to face the grief that accompanies the job. 'Unfortunately I think any female wanting to commentate is still going to ask themselves do they really want the hassle of pushing themselves to reach that level? To be slagged off. Because even if they're excellent they will still be slagged off by a large proportion of the viewing public. Do they want that in their life? Sadly that is going to be an issue for them and it will take someone with very thick skin to do that.'

Working to change that fact is Shelley Alexander, BBC Editorial Lead for Women's Sport and in charge of the BBC Sport outreach programme to find new talent. Shelley remembers being 'thrilled' on first meeting Jacqui and excited about her potential after she sent in some non-league commentary she had done for Radio Leeds. But what followed shocked even Shelley, a stalwart of the football industry. 'We knew it would be a big moment for football and the BBC but we were knocked sideways by the intensity of the scrutiny and unwarranted criticism that Jacqui's commentary received,' she tells me. 'It not only had a significant impact on Jacqui's professional development but I saw first-hand the chilling effect it had on the ambitions of other women to follow in Jacqui's footsteps.'

Shelley has since worked on a number of BBC schemes to encourage new talent, and one of these led to a specific initiative aimed at encouraging young women through regional opportunities, Women in Local Radio Sport (WIRLS). 'These women commentators are still learning their trade and, just like Jacqui Oatley in her early days, they need to be nurtured and given the opportunity out of the limelight to progress, but there is no doubt that I am excited for the future. These WIRLS have not been pitched straight into commentating – they are learning the basic skills of sports reporting and the hope is that eventually several of them will progress to become commentators in the future, and their visibility in the meantime does inspire other young women to consider this career.' We certainly need them, and not just in football. It's so rare to hear a woman commentating on any sport. British gymnastics coach Christine Still commentates on men's gymnastics as well as women's, but you'd be hard-pressed to name many female commentators across other sports. Alison Mitchell flies the flag for women in cricket, Sara Orchard has done the same in rugby, Katherine Merry commentates on IPC championships – but there are no female commentators, for example, in able-bodied athletics despite it being a sport for men and women.

It will take a few years, but one of the women on Shelley's scheme could just end up being the next female commentator on *Match of the Day*. If that happened, would we ever accept them? Is the female vocal register a non-starter for sports fans? Shelley cuts through the prejudice. 'What they have to all achieve to make it to the top of the game is consistent, measured delivery to achieve accuracy, clarity and colour – painting those match pictures and bringing the excitement and passion of a football match. This applies most significantly to that marvellous moment when a goal is scored. It is here that a commentator faces a formidable challenge – how to bring all the thrill and information about the goal while preventing their voice from rising too much. This is a skill that men and women commentators must learn equally, and it is only by training and experience that they can perfect it.'

What's important about Shelley's analysis is that it doesn't refer to the register or pitch of a person's voice. It is not about which note they come out with, it's about how controlled they are in their delivery, and that control is most evident in calling a goal, a try, a strike, a match-winning point. The skill of a commentator is in conveying the excitement of the moment, but with enough authority and restraint to guide the viewer or listener through the events. It is about *how* a voice is employed, not which note it hits. Crucially, that makes the gender of the commentator irrelevant.

Thankfully, we are making inroads. In 2013 the BBC's Charlotte Green was the first woman to read out the football results on the radio, and Rebecca Lowe – now stateside at NBC – became the first woman to host an FA Cup final. In 2014 former England cricketer Isa Guha became the first female summarizer on *Test Match Special*, while my colleague Amy Lawrence and England and Chelsea striker Eniola Aluko were the first women to feature as *Match of the Day* pundits, albeit on the offshoot *MOTD2 Extra*. Meanwhile in a little patch of Hertfordshire, Emma Saunders – a BBC journalist – has been making inroads as a stadium announcer for Watford FC's

Premier League campaign, and the UK even has its own all-female podcast in *The Offside Rule Podcast (We Get It!)*, featuring Hayley McQueen, Lynsey Hooper and Kait Borsay.

Many of these women do not have elite sporting careers on their CVs; they are just ordinary women who happen to feel passionately about sport, and who have the talent, the voice and the determination to convey it. They probably don't think of themselves as beacons of change, but for the young girls watching their presence will be significant, and inspirational. And for the sceptics, their success further normalizes women having a voice in sport – whether that's pursuing a career path, or simply giving a fan's view about football.

Over in the US, the long-time absence of authentic female voices in sports media led to a much more vocal response from women. In September 2014, at the height of the NFL's domestic violence crisis, Fox Sports presenter Katie Nolan launched a video blog criticizing her own industry – and her employer – for the part it plays in supporting a misogynistic culture in sport. 'Women in sports TV are allowed to read headlines, patrol sidelines and generally facilitate conversation for their male colleagues,' said Nolan in a vlog that attracted over 370,000 views. 'And, while the [sports journalists] Stephen A. Smiths, Mike Cairns, Dan Patricks and Keith Olbermanns of the world get to weigh in on the issues of the day, we just smile, and throw to commercial. A lot of people like to justify the role of women in sports media by saying, "Well, they've never played the game, so they aren't qualified to speak about it." Because God forbid someone misspeak about The Game. But topics like domestic violence, and racism and corruption? Let's let [commentator] Boomer [Esiason] handle those between downs. It's time for the conversation to change. Or at least those participating in the conversation. It's time for women to have a seat at the big-boy table. And not just as a gimmick or a concept but just a person who happens to have breasts offering their opinion on the sports they love and the topics they know.' Katie's pay-off line was perhaps the most revealing as she challenged the industry, and her own employer, to improve: 'Because the truth is the NFL will never respect women and their opinions as long as the media it answers to doesn't. I'm ready when you are, Fox.'[34]

Echoing Katie's words came the launch of an all-female-line-up sports show on CBS Sport, *We Need To Talk*. While the title has been panned, the show – which is produced and directed by an all-female staff – is an inevitable result of widespread frustrations. Twelve high-profile women, including former Oakland Raiders CEO Amy Trask and world boxing champion Laila Ali (daughter of Muhammad Ali), debate the issues of the day across men and women's sport from a uniquely female angle. Emilie Deutsch, one of the show's coordinating producers, told *Sports Illustrated* why the programme was a no-brainer. 'I want this show to succeed for all these little girls across the country who sit and watch baseball games with their Dads and Moms and want to get into this business and have been – and I choose these words carefully – relegated to three minutes during a football game . . . It's time for women to have a real platform.'[35] I find it telling how often conversations about these issues lead to thoughts about how they will affect the next generation. As a mum, I am determined that my own daughter will never experience this kind of nonsense. That she will never view sport as a no-go area that she cannot talk about, participate in, or pursue a career in.

Because, frankly, it's this kind of stuff that puts women off. Women who might otherwise be football fans, but instead prefer to steer clear. Like my friend Sophie Loi-Shaw, who grew up loving Arsenal, wearing the shirt and singing the songs, but eventually downed tools out of sheer frustration. Unexpectedly, during the 2014 World Cup in Brazil Sophie called me excitedly to say how much she was loving the football. 'I'd forgotten how much I actually *liked* football,' she said. 'It's brilliant, isn't it? The stuff on the actual pitch. It's just all the other bollocks that I hate. The money, the media, the bigotry. If only all that could go away and we could just enjoy the football. Like the Olympics. Why can't football be more like the Olympics?'

The thing is, it can! There's no reason why we all have to carry on with the blokey singing, and the trying to fit in, and the nervously hoping no one will notice that there's a woman at the game, or the blushing when they do, or putting up with the dumb rape chants, or the stupid football marketing departments who believe that women *will only buy* their club shirt if it is reproduced in the same candyfloss pink that every other football club has selected for their female fans. Or the World Cup widow email spam, or the offside-rule handbag and shoe shopping analogies. Enough! Women like football. Women like sport. And we don't want to change any of the good stuff about it, it's just that some of us would quite like to change the terrible stuff. You know, the really embarrassing stuff that we never want our daughters or sons to hear. We just want to make it nicer for all of us. By adding our voices – our presence – we can own our own sporting space, our own sporting voice. And that can sound however we want it to. Whether that means shrieking in our highest register as the goals go flying in, opining on defensive play, or just having a natter about Gary Lineker's naff new facial hair. It's all valid.

The opportunity to define our own female voice in sport is now. To be sports fans in the way that we want to be – hell, maybe we don't want to memorize the entire weekend's results for all four professional football leagues; maybe it's OK just to enjoy the game and not have to *prove* our fandom. Maybe we'll even bring some men along with us on the way; they might just find it refreshing. In the twenty-first century women should be strong enough and smart enough to trust in our own authenticity. To enjoy the sound of our voice, and to use it collectively to claim sport as a conversation for us to join in with: on the terraces, in the pubs and cafes, and certainly over the airwaves.

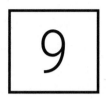

Women's sport: changing the game

Clare Balding said it first: 2015 would be the year that changes sport for women and girls. It certainly felt that way; from the US women's World Cup win prompting President Obama to say, 'Playing like a girl means you're a badass,' to Australian jockey Michelle Payne becoming an overnight sensation in winning the Melbourne Cup and then telling the misogynists in horse racing to 'get stuffed'. England's women cricketers turned professional and the ECB revealed plans to launch the very first organized domestic league; Maggie Alphonsi – England's greatest-ever female rugby star – became the first female pundit at a men's rugby World Cup, and in tennis, tickets for the women's US Open final sold out before the men's for the very first time, thanks to Serena Williams (even though, in the end, she didn't make the final). Amid the revolution, though, America's UFC Bantamweight Champion Ronda Rousey has arguably provided the greatest shake-up of all.

I first heard about Ronda early in 2015 at a talk I gave as part of the Pioneers in Sport forum, a venture aimed at breathing new life into a very old order. In the audience was David

Allen, vice president of the Ultimate Fighting Championship, and as he left he told me the story of a female fighter whose pay-per-view fights were outselling the men. I couldn't quite believe it. Ronda, he said, was something special. Within six months everyone knew her name. She was on every US TV station, every magazine cover, she even had a porn parody named after her: Ronda ArouseMe. Soon there was an autobiography out – written by her sports journalist sister – and she was starring in blockbuster Hollywood movies like *Entourage*. Less than five years after UFC president Dana White said women would never be allowed to compete in the world's ultimate mixed martial arts fighting championship, Ronda is officially his biggest earner, his greatest star – male or female.

Ronda's entry into the big time has been like a whirlwind – reinventing the rules for female athletes. She is frequently lusted over as a sex symbol, and it's true she has done her fair share of photo shoots in bikinis. But most of the time she's not interested in playing pretty girl. She never wears make-up in the ring. She's there to do business, hair tied back, muscles primed, face red with exertion, sometimes gruesomely bloodied. Even when she ventured into Carl's Jr. territory (a US fast-food chain with a history of unbelievably sexual adverts) she managed to rewrite the script, snarling at the breakfast sandwich, interspersed with grainy footage of her in the ring. She has the body of a fighter: thick torso, muscly arms, powerful legs. She has the mouth of a fighter too, trash-talking boxer Floyd Mayweather. Floyd tried to hit back with some weak insults, pretending he'd never heard of her, and then boasting about how much more money he makes. But every time Floyd speaks he reminds us how smart Ronda is. I love her war of words with him: 'I wonder how Floyd feels being beat by a woman for once,' she said, referring to his domestic violence charges after she beat him to the title of ESPY best fighter award. Or, 'He said, "When you make $300 million a night, then you can give me a call." . . . I did the math and I think I actually make two to three times more than he does per second. So when he learns to read and write, he can text me.' Despite the animosity, after Ronda got knocked out by Holly Holm in the fight that shocked the world, Floyd surprised everyone by defending her from the trolls revelling in her defeat. Perhaps she's earned respect in even the most unlikely of corners.

Such has Ronda's impact been on mainstream culture that Beyoncé incorporated a video recording of her 'do-nothing bitch' speech into her own concert. Watching the YouTube footage, it's incredibly powerful to hear Ronda's voice booming out to thousands in the crowd, her words illuminated across the stage, as the introduction for Beyoncé's song 'Diva'. The biggest pop star on the planet referencing women's sport in her show? That's unprecedented. But then so too, perhaps, is Ronda's rhetoric. 'I think it's hilarious if people say that my body looks masculine,' said Ronda in the now-infamous speech. 'I'm like, "Listen, just because my body was developed for a purpose other than fucking millionaires doesn't mean it's masculine." I think it's femininely badass as fuck because there's not a single muscle on my body that isn't for a purpose. Because I'm not a do-nothing bitch.' The phrase was immortalized on a T-shirt, a proportion of the price going towards Didi Hirsch Mental Health Services, a charity in southern California. Typical Ronda: cashing in on her celebrity, and doing a good thing at the same time.

For all of these reasons Ronda has been dubbed the biggest feminist in sport, having successfully fought for the prefix 'women's' to be removed from UFC titles and ring introductions – the first sport ever to do so. 'I think we need to do whatever we can to take the word "woman" out of it,' she said ahead of a fight in Melbourne. 'I don't hear people saying, "men's this, men's that" at the men's press conference. People are here today not because they love women, but because they love fighters. We're fighters. It's not the "women's UFC bantamweight"; I'm the bantamweight champion, she's the strong weight champion, and these people are here because they love fights.' Meanwhile she's called out the sexist interviewers who focus on her private life, she embraces her body – including her cauliflower ears – and she's criticized women like Kim Kardashian for selling Skechers trainers to teenage girls off the back of her rise to fame via a leaked sex tape.

But not everyone is a fan. Her autobiography describes her beating a former boyfriend after she discovered he had been taking naked photos of her in secret. Ronda claims he wouldn't let her leave the house, she felt trapped and that's why she hit him. Others say she is a hypocrite for flagging up Floyd's domestic violence record when she has committed her own offences. She drew staunch criticism from the trans community after saying transgender UFC fighter Fallon Fox should not be allowed to fight women because of a perceived, albeit scientifically unproven, advantage. She competes in a sport more violent than boxing. And her view on sport's gender pay gap is unsympathetic to many female athletes whose events attract less commercial investment than their male counterparts. 'I think that how much you get paid should have something to do with how much money you bring in,' said Ronda ahead of a press conference in Australia. 'I'm the highest paid UFC fighter not because Dana and Lorenzo wanted to do something nice for the ladeez; they do it because I bring in the most money. And I think that the money they make should be proportionate to the money they bring in.'

On the face of it she's right, of course. But Ronda fails to mention the many centuries of discrimination, barriers and oppression faced by women who tried to play sport. The fact is that sport has always been a feminist issue, whether sportswomen wish to acknowledge it or not.

And that's where Serena Williams swooped in and blew us all away with a powerful speech on winning the *Sports Illustrated* Sportsperson of the Year award in 2015. An athlete like Serena could opt for a quiet life and decide not to use her platform of influence as a voice for change. Few sportspeople – men or women – do. But, in the vein of Ronda, Serena is not like other athletes. She is fearless, and heroic. And she chose to use her moment in the limelight to send a powerful message to those who routinely ignore and undermine the achievements of sportswomen, and in particular women of colour.

Incredibly, Serena was the first sportswoman to win the *SI* award in three decades, and the first ever to win it outright as an individual. Brilliantly, she highlighted this fact in her winning speech. And she didn't sugar coat the truth about just how hard she's had to fight for recognition. 'I've had people look down on me, put me down because I didn't look like them – I look stronger,' she said. 'I've had people look past me because of the colour of my skin, I've had people overlook me because I was a woman, I've had critics say I [would] never win another

Grand Slam when I was only at number seven – and here I stand today with twenty-one Grand Slam titles, and I'm still going.'

At the end of the speech she quoted the poet Maya Angelou, selecting stanzas from 'Still I Rise' which were so charged with the history of slavery and discrimination that listening to her recite the words out loud made me weep. Your insults, she seems to say, are as old as the hills, steeped in slavery and America's struggle with the civil rights movement. Because Serena's success, as she sees it, connects directly with the effort to bring women of colour out of oppression. In a world where celebrities are expected to say the most marketable things, the lines that fit in with PR plans, mass appeal and profit, Serena is brutally honest.

She didn't read out Maya Angelou's stanza about black female sexuality being an affront to white society, but she didn't need to. She'd already posed on the front cover of *Sports Illustrated*, one bare leg casually slung over the armrest of a mock throne, to cries of 'prostitute' in the US national media. She didn't need to say it, but the subtext was clear: the rules of this game are set so that she cannot possibly win. One minute she is accused of being so masculine that her body provides her with an unfair advantage over her opponents, the next she is so sexually female she apparently looks more like a sex worker than the world's greatest-ever female tennis star.

We can only be grateful that Serena has chosen to pick up this mantle. Sport is a vital platform for change. Why else did US sprinters Tommie Smith and John Carlos give the black power salute at the 1968 Olympic Games? The United Nations have declared that sport will play a leading role in the fight for gender equality in the twenty-first century. If every athlete could use their voice to create change the world would be a better place. Clare Balding agrees. 'Women's sport helps break down a lot of barriers for women in other areas. Sport in schools was the beginning of physical freedom for women and it is terribly important still, particularly for women in the Middle East. If you're not allowed to run or sweat in public, that's part of your freedom that's being eroded, but if you are allowed to go to the Olympics then I think it's massive. It's part of the catalyst for social change. It's to do with being allowed to be judged on your talent, but also it's to do with clothing. If you look back at British history, women being allowed to play sport in schools meant they could change their clothing. They couldn't be running around in their long skirts and corsets.'

Clare's right to point to history. Because rewriting our history is an important part of all this. Women's sporting achievements have long been absent from the history books. So while I learned about the suffragettes at school, I had no idea that the real reason there is no female Wayne Rooney banking £300K a week is because women's football was banned in this country from 1921 to 1971. Prior to the ban 53,000 people turned up to watch women play football at Goodison Park in 1920. Throughout history, right into the twenty-first century, women have repeatedly been prevented from taking part in sport. And I'm not just talking about developing countries. Right here in the west we have only just secured a spot for women ski jumpers to compete in the Winter Olympics because the president of the FIS, Gian Franco Kasper, was still arguing that the sport was medically dangerous for wombs. Meanwhile in the UK just two statues of sportswomen are on public display: tennis player Dorothy Round and pentathlete Mary Peters. And in 2013 the

Royal Mail celebrated 150 years of football with a series of stamps of exclusively male footballers.

Serena has told us before that she stands on the shoulders of other women's achievements, but most of us probably have no idea just how many centuries the fight for women's sport spans. It is virtually unknown that the Heraean Games of Ancient Greece were the Olympic equivalent for women, or that in Sparta women were encouraged to wrestle, or that in medieval England nuns played cricket, or that Anne Boleyn was watching tennis the day she was arrested and taken to the Tower, or that Mary, Queen of Scots was a talented golfer. Meanwhile, in the twentieth century, legendary fashion designer Coco Chanel tore up fashion rules as a result of being influenced by tennis and sportswear design in her now-iconic couture.

We are often told that sport is unnatural for women, that there is no history of women participating, or even being interested in sport – unlike men. But while the barriers have been huge, women still sought to break them. And while we're reviewing our past, we should probably rewrite our present too, celebrating the multiple female mega celebrities who love sport – from Mary J. Blige's passion for running, to Helen Mirren's support for women's football. The more we can do to normalize women's relationship with sport, the better chance we have for change.

In redefining the limits of women's sport, one of the most exciting opportunities for a level playing field lies in sports where women can compete against men. And in 2015 there was no better example of that than Michelle Payne's historic win at the Melbourne Cup, Australia's first-ever win from a female jockey in a major race. Michelle used the exposure to make her point about female jockeys being equal to men – when they are lucky enough to be properly supported. But her success wasn't an isolated moment. Just a few months before, a trio of women jockeys had won the Shergar Cup, racing's team riding event at Ascot, Emma-Jayne Wilson, Sammy Jo Bell and Hayley Turner blowing away the male competition. Meanwhile Katie Walsh, younger sister of the legendary Ruby Walsh, became only the third woman to win the Irish Grand National. For Katie, the opportunity to compete against men is to be relished. 'That's what's unique in horse racing, I can take on a level playing field,' Katie told me. 'It's great to have that uniqueness. It's everyone for their own out there, it's not like women's tennis or women's golf, we're all there together. You're seen as good as the next person on the day – you just have to produce it. I think it's great, I love that we can do that.

'Horse racing is not just about the jockey, it's about the horse. And no matter how successful you are, if I get up on a horse and it's a way better horse than a horse that Ruby might get up on, Ruby's not going to win just because he's Ruby Walsh. I would probably win if I was on the better horse.'

It's getting the rides that remains the challenge for women jockeys, with Katie hearing first hand just how prejudiced some can be in the sport when she interviewed British Race School tutor Michael Tebbutt in a special report for the BBC, in which he denigrated female jockeys as lacking in physical and mental strength compared to their male counterparts. Women in Racing, an organization for which Katie is an ambassador, were outraged. Sally Rowley-Williams, founder and chair, explained why Michael's words could not be taken as a joke – particularly when female jockeys still face an uphill struggle to be given the same opportunities as men. 'There hasn't yet been a big owner hiring a female jockey on a retainer. Not one, over the flat, or the jumps. And that makes things very difficult for female jockeys because they're not getting the best rides. There's a lot of work to do around changing hearts and minds.'

Hopefully the tale of Victoria Pendleton, the two-time Olympic gold medallist in cycling turned amateur jockey, is helping to shine a light on the potential of female jockeys. Certainly, the sport is in flux. There are more female trainers than ever, and the British Horseracing Authority is the first major sports board to announce a 50 per cent gender split in its directors.

All good progress, but until the opportunities are there across the board, the salaries are never going to match the men's. Ultimately, what Ronda – and others – need to understand is that when women aren't paid the same as men in sport, it's not because they don't earn it, it's more often than not because their sport hasn't benefited from decades – centuries – of privilege, development and investment. Most sports fans are pretty comfortable with the idea that Wayne Rooney earns more than England captain Steph Houghton, because there is more money in men's football and so the wages reflect that. When women's sport attracts greater investment, goes the argument, then sportswomen will receive higher salaries. Except that once you start to get down and dirty with the figures, it's not so easy to sit comfortably with this logic. For example, how can it be right that the US women's team won the Women's World Cup, destroyed the men's US World Cup viewing figures, and were given a cheque for $2m., while the men's US team went out in the knockout stages the summer before and earned themselves

$8m.? You can talk about market forces until you're blue in the face, but that just doesn't add up.

It's clear, then, that we need a different approach. If we are going to have a sensible discussion about pay and women's sport we need to understand that the market forces cannot be our starting point. We need more imagination than that. Helena Morrissey, founder of the 30% Club and CEO of Newton Investment Management, literally threw the spreadsheet out of the window when she began to invest in women's sport. I love the way she tells the story of some hapless agency bringing her the same old boring male sports investment opportunities, 'the usual thing of buying a rugby shirt for a vast sum of money. We weren't exactly bowled over,' she says, drily.[36] Most corporates are falling over themselves to get their names on the shirts of the male sporting elite. Not Helena: she finds it pointless. Because how much financial return do you actually get after paying out all that cash? Instead she demanded that the agency look into a sport where her investment would make a real difference. They came back with the story of the women's Boat Race, two penniless teams with no profile and no exposure. Helena listened, and jumped at the chance. Thirty thousand pounds later and she had secured both Oxford and Cambridge's women's teams. But rather than sit back and watch what might happen next, she waded right into the heart of the action.

On hearing that the women had never been allowed to compete on the Thames tideway, unlike their male peers, she marched down to the various deans' offices and demanded to know why. 'And they would harrumph and look down, shuffle from one leg to another,' she grins, 'and then someone said to me: "You know that's the question you're not really supposed to ask?"' But the race location was duly changed. Then she asked why the BBC couldn't show it live alongside the men, and despite some quibbling about the practicalities of getting the camera back to the start line in time, they also caved. Before long Clare Balding had quit the Grand National so she could host this now-historic event live on the BBC, and suddenly the women's Boat Race went from total and utter obscurity to front-page news, the biggest sports story of the week. Better still, for Helena, Newton Investment Management became a household name, proving that the 0.4 per cent of sponsorship that goes towards women's sport in the UK is not only appalling, embarrassing and archaic, but also grossly short-sighted. Helena tells me that Repucom estimated her financial return at tenfold the original investment. That seems like a pretty smart piece of business to me. The challenge is, as Helena brightly puts it, that women's sport requires a new way of thinking, 'a vision, not a spreadsheet, because women's sport requires you to create something, to campaign, not just sit in a corner.'

Helena's message is one that I've tried to relay to everyone who will listen. For me it is the key to solving this dilemma of how to convince investors to put assets into women's sport. Helena's words sum up the excitement of an evolving sector, the opportunities that brings, and the chance to be actively involved, actively shaping history. By contrast, sticking a corporate name on the shirt of a men's team seems a pretty passive investment.

The wonderful thing about women's sport is that most of those involved in it are not looking at the spreadsheet first and foremost. Often, they don't even care about the money – they wouldn't be in it if they did. They're involved because they're passionate and committed, and that's a pretty special workforce to harness. These are people who want what Helena's talking about: a smart approach, a structure that will grow and develop their sport, a plan that leads to money, but first relies on ingenuity over investment. Because while men's sport can plough pounds into the women's game and change individual lives, that alone will never be enough to truly change women's sport forever.

After an incredible tournament for England's female footballers at the 2015 World Cup, including a record two million viewers for matches that she presented on the BBC, Jacqui Oatley is one of those stalwarts desperate for the sport to finally realize its marketing and investment potential. She believes those elements are key in order to secure its long-term existence. 'As long as women's football is not self-funding there's always a concern that the bubble could burst and we could go back to the way it was before,' she says. 'Maybe not players paying to play, but you've always got to worry it might go back to being semi-pro.'

In a column for *Glamour* magazine, she urged women to get off their sofas and actually go to watch live women's sport. If you believe in it, she argued, then you must actively support it. 'We still don't have a culture of people going to watch women's football so you're trying to get people to change their social recreational habits and that won't happen overnight,' she tells me. 'But I still think a huge amount can be done from a marketing point of view. It's becoming a spectator sport on the TV because we're getting great viewing figures, but we need people to go to the games and know where to get tickets.' To that end, Jacqui is forever tweeting about kick-off times, where to buy tickets, prices and transport. She believes, as England and

Chelsea striker Eniola Aluko and others do too, that more needs to be done. Best of all, she's bubbling over with solutions. 'It's not just about media coverage, the FA still put money into the Women's Super League – they are literally paying clubs to exist which a lot of people don't quite realize. They pay £70K to each club in WSL1 [core funding] which the clubs have to match, and £35K to WSL2. But it has to be self-sustaining and that's why I get the bee in my bonnet about marketing and the clubs not doing enough. I don't think there's enough initiative and creativity. They don't use the men's Twitter feed enough or send a male player like John Terry down to [Chelsea ladies' ground] Staines to sign autographs. A lot of Chelsea fans don't even know where the women play. It's frustrating. A lot needs to be done to drive traffic through the turnstiles; it can be done, but it's not happening.'

It still feels as though some of the best solutions lie outside the sports industry. Like the phenomenal poster campaign that went viral during the World Cup following Lucy Bronze's winning strike to take England through to the semi-finals. '2015: the year boys all over England score goals in their gardens, whilst pretending they're called Lucy', it read. Genius. The campaign worked so well because it told us something new about women's sport. It didn't bang on about women's sport being a purer, more virtuous, morally superior version of the men's game – which is often how women's sport is cloyingly described. Instead it just told us: this is the coolest thing, and even the opposite sex think so. Because they really do. Like the boys in Spike Lee's film pretending to be Mo'ne Davis, the campaign tapped into a very modern way of thinking. Women's sport is getting big, and everyone wants to be a part of it.

Thank goodness, then, that we have people like Jacqui on the case. Clare Balding aside, I honestly can't think of another TV presenter who rolls their sleeves up to promote women's sport quite like Jacqui does. Why does she do it? 'Injustice, I absolutely hate injustice,' she tells me. 'Which sounds a bit grand when you're talking about football. But I do. For example, look at [England star] Kelly Smith, look at the talent she has got. And she had to go to America to get the recognition she deserves, to play at a certain standard. What a shame she couldn't play more in this country to that standard. When she played for Arsenal Ladies she'd play in front of crowds of eighty people. That was standard! That's injustice, to me. She could probably walk down the street in this country and most people would not know she is Kelly Smith, the greatest female player this country's ever had. That annoys me. I get so frustrated by that. And that's gone now. We've seen the best of her now. Look at Rachel Yankey who pretended to be a boy called Ray just so she could play! You just hope the new generation gets a better deal. Look at the recognition Fran Kirby got for scoring one goal at the World Cup, and she's on a good wage and doesn't have to work now; you just hope it continues.'

If the sports media have historically been given a kicking for not supporting women's sport – in 2013 just 2 per cent of national newspaper sports pages carried women's sport – women's magazines get a harder time still. Frequently characterized as obsessed with beauty, fashion and sex, they have hitherto been reluctant to change their attitude towards sport. That is, until *Glamour* editor Jo Elvin took a huge leap and began flying the flag for change. At the start of 2015 *Glamour* launched a major campaign, 'Say No To Sexism In Sport'.

I went to meet Jo at *Glamour*'s offices off Regent Street, just as London Fashion Week was in full flow. Her bright corner office was covered in designer clothes and bags, as immaculately turned-out women sashayed between desks carrying coffee. But Jo couldn't have been more down to earth. As someone who hated sport at school, she told me how she was one of those 'grumpy people' who had dreaded the arrival of the London Olympic Games, and booked a holiday to flee the capital. 'But I ended up watching it on TV every night,' she laughs. 'Watching Jessica Ennis, Mo Farah, and there's me crying in front of the TV. I'm not even British! I'm Australian! Why do I care about Team GB? And I remember feeling, knowing, that the minute it was all over women's sport would get relegated back to low profile. No profile. And I don't know why but that just really annoyed me.' Eighteen months later, and a story came out about England footballer Fara Williams having been homeless at the height of her career. 'That just made me so angry,' says Jo now. 'We had internal collective conversations about it, and we decided to do something about it. We're the biggest-selling women's magazine, and we hadn't really concentrated on sport that much until the Olympics. We've always had a Sports-woman of the Year but we felt we could build on that. Because there was me complaining about how it wasn't covered, but I knew I was one of the people who hadn't covered it.'

Jo cites a 'huge feminist shift' in the last five years in terms of how women's magazines cover issues such as body image and exercise, and a sports campaign seemed a logical extension of that. Still, I admire Jo hugely for taking what would at the time have been perceived as a big risk. After all, if women really don't like sport, then how would they react to seeing it taking up space in pages where they would expect to see beauty and fashion? What took the team aback was the positive response from their readers. 'We've done campaigns before, but we've never had a response like this. It has shown me that most of our readers are into some kind of sport or fitness. We had letters saying, "Thank you so much for covering this, I've been made to feel unfeminine because I like football."' Stories like Jo's and Helena's prove that taking what are perceived to be business risks around women's sport in fact often pays off, and triumphantly at that. They are pioneers for change, but I hope others will take heart from their experiences and form a stampede towards women's sport.

As part of its commitment *Glamour* now covers women's sport in every issue, and has launched its own women's sport awards to rival the BBC Sports Personality ones that have so often been panned for failing to recognize the breadth and depth of women's sporting talent.

But if coverage is on the up, and corporate investors are finally rethinking their approach, what about the fans? The bums on seats that form such a critical part of the equation? *Glamour* is doing its bit to promote women's sport to women, but should men also be interested? Whenever the debate comes up, the popular view seems to be that women should be the ones to change the status quo. Because why be a sofa feminist? Go out and support a women's team, for God's sake! But why wouldn't we want men to watch women's sport too? Why wouldn't we encourage all existing sports fans to watch women's sport, and not just clamour for women to do so?

Sadly, for the men who do follow women's sport it's not always the easiest ride. Society has so little belief in women's sport that people can't fathom why a man would be interested. But they are! Football journalist Tony Leighton has been covering the women's game for years, and now a new generation is joining him. Kieran Theivam started off writing about Watford for his local newspaper, but a chance interview with England's star striker Kelly Smith piqued his interest in the women's game. 'For me watching women's football is an escape from what men's football has turned into,' he says. 'I'm a bit of an old git, but Watford used to be about focusing on academy players. This season [2014/15] going into the Premier League we've spent loads of money and signed thirteen players. People are becoming disgruntled with men's sport and are turning to women and minority sports. As a journalist I find that the women are more open, intelligent, articulate and interesting than many of the male footballers I've ever interviewed.'

Kieran launched England's first-ever women's football podcast in 2013. 'I've never done it for the money. I do it because I enjoy it. I won't deny it's hard work – I finish work at 6 p.m. and most evenings I'm working on podcasts and articles; it takes up a lot of my time but I wouldn't have it any other way.' If anything, Kieran is out of pocket when he covers the sport; he paid his own expenses to attend the World Cup in Canada, and didn't earn a penny for the articles he wrote out there. 'Some people think I'm mad,' he shrugs.

I love Kieran's passion for the game, and I respect his knowledge. And so I can't help but feel angry when he shyly tells me that, as a young man in his early thirties, he is embarrassed by occasional jokes and insinuations about why he is interviewing a certain female player, or why he might be covering a match where teenage girls are on the pitch. 'It's only people joking around,' he says quietly, 'but it's not a nice position to be in. I know some male supporters who are worried about going to watch the sport because of it.'

Why are some women doing to men what has been done to us for so long? I had years of those sorts of comments as a sports journalist. Readers would write in to our newspaper and claim that I based my man of the match award verdicts on the players with the sexiest legs. Or there would be the blog comments about how I was only doing my job because I wanted to marry a footballer.

In this brave new world of supporting women's sport I think we need to do away with these kinds of attitude, and embrace male engagement. Kieran also wishes more women would support the women's game. 'I know a lot of female supporters who follow Watford men's team, but would never watch the women. There's this perception out there that it's just men who have a dim view of the game, but it's women too.' And it's not just the fans who have a problem with it. He attends home games at Arsenal Ladies' Borehamwood ground most weeks, and says the press box is largely occupied by men. He has a point. I've spoken to several female sports journalists who are reluctant to cover women's sport for fear of being pigeonholed.

Chris Scott, a former women's sport blogger now working in the industry, tells me, 'You need men supporting women's sport to show it's not a minority sport, it's not a special interest group.' Uniquely, Chris grew up surrounded by women who were more sporty than the men he knew. 'Naively, I didn't actually realize there was an issue [with gender inequality in sport] at the time, probably because there was a far greater number of competent sportswomen in our friendship group than sportsmen. It was normal for me. And that's why I find it easy to say that women's sport should have an equal platform to men, equal funding, equal coverage, equal engagement. When people disagree I find it very frustrating because I've never thought differently. It makes me want to bang my head on the table.' Chris's experience proves that our environment goes a long way towards forming our attitudes about women's sport. And that, sometimes, different environments will throw up unexpected outcomes.

It was with interest, then, that I spoke to Hadassah, a mother of four from the Orthodox Jewish community in Stamford Hill, North London – a close-knit, traditional community with specific cultural requirements around gender roles. I was intrigued to hear from a friend that in Charedi schools girls are encouraged to do regular PE lessons, albeit in modest, long-sleeved attire. By contrast, as Hadassah explained it to me, Charedi boys are most at risk from inactivity because their purpose is defined as studying the Torah as much as possible. 'The Charedi lifestyle is generally sedentary,' says Hadassah, 'and sport hasn't necessarily been encouraged because of an association with glamorizing the body and image worshipping.' But as diabetes and obesity rates rose in the community a decided shift began to take place. 'Sport and exercise is now beginning to be understood as something to do for health reasons – a commandment in the Torah. I remember speaking to a woman running a community group ten years ago who told me, "Sport is not for us, my mother always told me that we get our exercise by scrubbing the kitchen counter." But these days her group does offer exercise. It's as much recognized for mental health benefits as anything else.'

Still, sport remains a largely alien concept in the community. Despite its proximity to the site of the Olympic Park, Hadassah says that most of the North London Charedi do not access mainstream newspapers, radio or television – and most had little, if any, involvement in the London 2012 Olympics. And while girls at school may be allowed a single weekly PE lesson, once they become women their focus is usually on managing the home, often while working part-time. 'The average family in our community has six children. That takes its toll on a woman's body,' says Hadassah. Attitudes for women are changing, though, with the opening of a Charedi fitness centre offering gender-segregated sessions, and an application for a community-use pool – two vital facilities for Charedi women to access single-gender swimming, netball and aerobics. Hadassah tells me of a friend who was recently walking along the River Lee when a woman living on a houseboat stuck her head out of the window to enquire whether the rabbi had ordered that women walk for exercise, because she had seen so many more women walking up and down in the last year. Hadassah laughs. 'You see? Things are really changing, even in our community.' She tells me she is lucky to have a husband who – hailing from Amsterdam – approves of cycling for women. Every Friday morning, when the children are at school, the couple wheel their bikes to a quiet spot on the river and cycle together.

I find it inspiring that even in some of the most traditional communities and cultures, women and girls are finding a path to sport and exercise. More than that, it is a treasured activity. How many couples in mainstream western culture go cycling together, or engage in sport or exercise together? I am envious of Hadassah's Friday mornings with her husband. In mainstream western culture women may encounter barriers, but we also have a lot of opportunities to access sport and exercise. It is important that we don't take these for granted.

Some of the most uplifting stories that I've come across this past year have hailed from the Middle East, where women and girls are making bold strides, often in cultures that are actively hostile to their engagement. Typically, the depressing stories have earned the most column inches: the Iran futsal captain, Niloufar Ardalan, prevented from travelling to the Asian championships because her husband refused to sign papers allowing her to renew her passport (a requirement under Iranian law); the laws that prevent women from watching football or volleyball in Iranian stadiums; and Saudi Arabia's proposal to host a men-only Olympic Games. But there have been a haul of triumphant stories too. The Iraqi women's cycling team bringing back a sack of medals from the Arab and Asian Championships; the 2016 FIFA U-17 Women's World Cup, held in Jordan, which stipulates quotas for female coaches and medics for the first time at a global tournament; or – further east, in Pakistan – the social media hashtag #GirlsAtDhabas used alongside video and images of women playing street cricket in a movement to openly defy societal norms. Then there was the young woman who completed a marathon in Afghanistan – the first ever to do so – running through the streets despite stares and, at times, abuse and violence, to send a message to others that women can achieve anything, that women are strong. Before the race, in Bamiyan, she had trained in her family's small backyard running around in circles, as it was deemed too unsafe for her to run in the streets without an escort. Those stories of determination, of positivity, aren't shared enough in our mainstream media. That's a shame because there is a lot we can learn from the achievements of women elsewhere, overcoming barriers, pursuing their passion, finding their joy.

My final interview for this book was with two female Iraqi football coaches. Thousands of miles away in Sulaymaniya province, northern Iraq, Intisar Nawaf and Sarab Hassan sat at a desk in the office of Spirit of Soccer, the charity that employs them, peering into the computer as we spoke over Skype. An interpreter nestled between their chairs. I was struck by the fact that despite being 3,000 miles apart in such very different cultures, here we were talking about football and feminism.

Sarab and Intisar told me that, like many girls growing up in Iraq, they were prevented from playing sport by their fathers who worried about their reputation. How then, I asked, was it possible that they had now come to pursue a career as football coaches? Their story takes us back to 2014 when ISIS began to attack the city of Jalawla, in eastern Iraq, home to Intisar and her family. As the shells rained down, people fled on foot. 'We took nothing with us, just our three children and my husband,' says Intisar. 'After we left our home I felt very depressed. Everything we had worked for, everything we had built over many years, we just had to leave it all behind. That was very hard. But in the end I decided that the safety of my family is all that matters, the sacrifice is nothing compared to that.'

Jalawla has since been liberated, but Intisar and her family are not able to return home. The city has become known internationally as a ghost town. 'We cannot go back home because our city is full of bombs and explosives. No one lives there now. It's just police. God willing we will be able to go home one day. After liberation I went back for a day just to see my house. Inside I found a box with an electrical heater that I did not recognize. It wasn't anything that belonged to me. I called the police. It was a bomb, disguised as a heater. It is not safe for us to go there.'

'We live in an environment full of war,' says Sarab, nodding and listing off three decades of conflict, from the Iraq–Iran war of the 1980s to the Gulf War, the invasion by Allied forces in 2003 – and now ISIS. The legacy of war is generations of traumatized children, thousands of whom have been left physically disabled by forgotten landmines. Many are living in camps for refugees and Internally Displaced People (IDP). The camps in Kurdistan have no running water, electricity or sanitation. The tents are old, and leak when it rains. The atmosphere is tense, families fighting for scarce resources.

It is the job of Sarab and Intisar to visit the camps and provide a precious few hours of fun with a ball, a fleeting moment of childhood. But the coaches have an added humanitarian role: educating the children about the dangers of explosive remnants of war. 'After ISIS attacked they left many landmines and explosives,' explains Sarab. 'It's especially dangerous for children because they like to play, they are curious, they like to pick things up. They are the ones most affected by these explosives. We tell them: never pick a toy up off the road, it could be a bomb.' According to the United Nations almost one million Iraqi children are affected by landmines and other unexploded devices. Intisar knows first hand how dangerous such devices are. She once watched a child pick up a bomb, mistaking it for a toy. It exploded in his face.

Their jobs as football coaches have changed their lives. Not only are they now able to engage with sport every day, and earn a living from it, but the status of being a paid coach with humanitarian responsibilities has made their work respectable in the eyes of those who might previously have questioned any affiliation with sport for a woman. 'We are in the middle of an economic crisis in Iraq, and we are working to bring in money,' says Sarab, explaining the change in attitude from her extended family. 'Plus it is humanitarian work, not only football. With the salary I earn I am able to support my parents, sisters and brothers – if they need it. Because I am successful at my work my husband, and society, are proud of me.'

Intisar tells me that she, too, is now the main breadwinner in the family as a result of the coaching job. When the family left their home in Jalawla, her husband left his shop behind too. It was a long time before he could find work again; he has since secured a job in a smaller shop but it is poorly paid. Spirit of Soccer provide Intisar with a regular salary, but they also helped the family move out of the refugee camp and into a rented house of their own. 'My husband supports the work I am doing,' she says, 'my children are happy and so proud of me. My daughter is always imitating me, pretending to be a coach; she says, "Now you sit down, and I'll be the coach." When I go to work in the morning my husband and my children help me to prepare my equipment. Me and my husband are working together to make our children's dreams come true, to make sure they go to school. We live in a male-centred society, and a tribal one. But none of that has stopped me working as a coach. I thank God every day that I am helping women and children. I always tell the families in the camp my story, that I am also an IDP.'

Just as with Rimla Akhtar's work at the Muslim Women's Sport Foundation in the UK, the key to Sarab and Intisar's success is that as women coaches they make it possible for girls to take part in sport. 'When I work people are always surprised that I am female,' says Sarab. 'But most of the families whose daughters we coach wholeheartedly accept us because we are female coaches. The situation would be very different if it was a man coaching their daughters; that would not be allowed. The girls are especially happy when they see us, when they see their coach is a woman. We tell the girls they have the same right to play sport as the boys. But sometimes the girls we meet are so shy they won't even move. Most of the time it is their very first experience of playing football.'

Then Sarab says something very special, something that goes to the heart of what this book is all about. 'I feel like those girls are in a closed circle that they cannot get out of,' she says, quietly. I know that she is talking about Iraqi society, but I can't help feeling that it applies to women and girls the world over. 'Through sport we make an outlet for them. In our society a girl needs confidence to achieve her goals, it's not only about football. Sometimes the girls feel shy to go after a ball, but we try to encourage them. We tell them, "If you are shy to chase a ball, how can you achieve your dreams?" Playing sport makes you feel free. It makes you feel like you can achieve anything.'

In my life I have been too shy to chase a ball. It sounds silly when you say it out loud, as an adult. But if you think of it another way, it's pretty serious. Because if women are too nervous to chase a ball, what does that say about us? What does that say about how inhibited we are, in our bodies, in our minds, in our freedom? I don't believe that every woman has to play sport in order to be happy, but I do believe every woman and girl on this planet should have the right to move their bodies freely and playfully, free from inhibition, judgement, oppression. In any way they want to. That's the key to our own liberation. And the sooner we crack it, the happier – and the more equal – we will all be.

Epilogue

So how do we create change in our own lives? I'm not talking diets, boot camps, or even joining a sports club. I'm talking about sustainable, incremental change. Change that is do-able, and change that makes us feel good – not overwhelmed with extra pressures to adopt a new lifestyle.

Sometimes it's just about making the tiniest adjustments in your brain, being open to new things. Like when my husband asked if I wanted a game of pool and, instead of running in the opposite direction as I usually would, terrified of being awful, I said yes. And so we played – and we laughed. We were both terrible, and my hands shook and wobbled inelegantly as the cue rested on my fingers, and I chipped the white up in the air, and missed the easiest of shots. 'We must be the worst sports journalist pool players ever,' I joked.

And then, something happened. Because I was having fun, I began to relax. The twenty years since I last played pool as a teenager floated away, and in my hands the cue took on a renewed purpose – and I potted a ball. I felt amazing! I punched the air! 'Are you trying to hustle me?' my husband asked, grinning. It was game on. Off we went, then, potting balls, missing balls, laughing and joking and enjoying ourselves together. Negotiating the edges of the green baize with my six-month pregnancy bump, I immediately thought of ten-times world champion snooker player Reanne Evans, an inspirational female figure battling for equality in her sport – who once won a world title while seven and a half months pregnant. How triumphant must she have felt that day? 'I did it for both of us,' she told me in early 2015, 'me and my daughter. It was two against one . . .'[37] In the end my husband's skills won over, and he potted the black while I still had three balls on the table. But it didn't matter. We'd played a game together. We'd been competitive together. And it had made us smile.

Writing this book helped the changes sink into my own brain. When my daughter asked me to run down the street with her, I stopped automatically saying, 'I can't because Mummy's got a baby in her tummy.' Instead I started saying, 'OK . . . race you!' Out of breath, hips sore, shopping bags bumping by my side, I lolloped along with her. We both laughed our heads off, and the baby was fine. Or we'd be in the park, Ella pedalling furiously on her bike with pink stabilizers, me lightly jogging alongside her in my winter boots, or chasing after her, racing in the wintry rain with my husband, the three of us grinning with delight. And each and every time I couldn't help but marvel at how physical activity brings such an unadulterated joy, unmatched by anything else.

Over the Christmas holidays I grew more and more aware of each time our family interacted with sport, as, for example, my husband sat watching Tottenham on the TV, while I, an Arsenal fan, quietly seethed in the background, and Ella delighted in this game of divided loyalties between her mum and dad. She would cosy up next to my husband and cheer her head off – occasionally for Arsenal, just to see the look on his face – and ask lots of questions. She wanted to understand what was happening, and she was most fascinated that adults had to follow rules, enforced by a referee handing out punishments to those who transgressed. 'I want to be a referee, Daddy,' she told my husband, 'or a goalkeeper.'

Conscious of how much men's sport is on TV, and of the lack of female role models for my daughter to follow, I took her down to our local athletics track where elite coach Christine Bowmaker, a rare example in her sport of a female coach, had invited us to watch her training sessions. Determined to make sure that my daughter has a better relationship with sport and her own body than I ever did, I was thrilled – and awestruck – as together we watched women and girls thundering around the bends of the indoor track, leaping onto boxes and into sandpits, and powering through circuits in the weights room. Outside we braved the December skies, and looked on as multiple gold-medallist Christine Ohuruogu ran 100m sprints in the cold air. 'That's Chrissy O.,' I told my daughter. 'She's won so many medals, and this is how she does it, with no one here to watch, no crowds, no TV cameras, just hard work, running around the track over and over again.' It's a lesson that sport teaches so well – how to achieve something, whether that's running or writing or reading. It takes practice and many days of hard work before you get the ticker-tape parade and the celebrations. I'm intrigued to see Ella looking on so concentratedly, spellbound.

Inside, Christine Bowmaker's young daughters are doing

their homework. 'Tell my girls they are allowed to play with Ella,' shouts Christine, stopwatch and notepad in hand, 'they won't dare otherwise.' We go inside, and there sits 'big' Ella, eight, and Indya, ten, diligently writing in their workbooks. I relay the message from their mum and the sisters look delighted to have been given a reprieve. Dressed in sports gear, with matching pink trainers, they tell us about their weekly activities – basketball, gymnastics, football, ballet, netball and, of course, a running session with their mum. My little Ella instantly idolizes them and wants to imitate their every move. Soon they are a gang. Watching Christine's group practise their block starts on the indoor track, the sisters show Ella how to crouch down for, 'On your marks, get set, go!' They demonstrate the different training drills to practise coordinating your steps out of the blocks – all mixed in with Stuck in the Mud, and It, for fun. When Ella gets tired, Indya carries her. They share snacks, and run about. All the while, Christine is glued to her sessions.

I think back to the hoo-ha over female coaches – particularly mothers – accused of not being able to do their jobs properly: Paralympic athlete Sophie Christenson having to defend her decision to employ a new mum as her coach, or the general consensus that mothers will always have to choose between family life and elite coaching, that there can never be a middle path. And I watch as Christine's children behave impeccably, not once disturbing their mother, while she gets on with flawlessly juggling the needs of a vast spectrum of athletes – from the world-class demands of Chrissy O., her up-and-coming younger sister Vicky, and the juniors just starting out in their careers. This job was made for a multitasker. You need your brain in a million places at once, and being a mother is perfect training for it. It is no surprise that Christine's coaching career is blossoming, despite the odds stacked against her.

While Ella plays with the girls I think about how powerful it is for us to be surrounded by all these active women. And I reflect on how easy it was to jump in our car, drive down the road, and find them. No, they're not on our TV as much as we'd all like, but these incredible female role models do exist, and there is a simple way of bringing them into my daughter's life. And it's worth it, because I can see how much she loves it. When we get home Ella doesn't stop talking about the girls and Christine; she wants to 'go running with them again, *please* mummy?'

Over the next few weeks I make sure Ella has proper running shoes and sports gear. She excitedly chooses a pair of light-blue trainers, 'They're just like [the film] *Frozen*, mummy!' and a pair of multicoloured running tights. In the trainer shop a sign reads, 'Kicks look great with dresses, for dancing in.' I smile. OK, so the message has its flaws, but it's a start. Even retailers are – slowly – changing. And my daughter loves wearing her trainers with a dress. Best of all, it means she can run super fast.

I need to do all of this because my daughter is four years old. She is not at school, she does not have PE lessons yet (good or bad), and most of the sporting opportunities I can find all begin at five or six. But kids make decisions about the world long before then. Even as toddlers they perceive and want to enact gendered roles. Unless we show even very young girls that sport and being physical is for them, there is a danger that they will already be dismissing it from the very earliest of ages. From the few things we have done together, I can already see the physical confidence growing in my own daughter: running, jumping, kicking a ball around the front room, wildly attempting hand-stands, dancing, play-fighting with her dad. I am happy to see her shine.

And then I remember myself. All of this is meaningless unless I am also part of the equation, unless I am also active. In timely fashion, US athlete Alysia Montaño, famous for compet-ing while eight months pregnant, tweets, 'Mommas 2 be need just as much support as someone training 4 the Olympics in quest of health & fitness in pregnancy.' Her message was in response to US Steeplechase champion Emma Coburn, who posted a picture of herself training for Rio alongside her nine-month-pregnant sister on the running machine. Mums need just as much support as someone training for the Olympics, I repeat to myself. Wow. Imagine if our health authorities saw things that way? What a change would be upon us.

Until then we have, mostly, ourselves to rely on. And each other. The last six months I have spent many hours at my desk writing about the importance of being active, while – frankly – being pretty inactive. Walking aside, I have been frightened to push my body in this pregnancy. I have lost my way, fallen off the wagon, and not really known how to get back on. I contact a fitness instructor who has been advising on the content of the book, and who specializes in antenatal and postnatal exercise. I ask her for some help – this time it's for me. I also join a preg-nancy yoga class, and I am thrilled when the teacher, Anjali, tells us all, 'Everyone says, "Oh you're pregnant, you must take it easy!" But they're wrong, you need to increase muscle tone, strengthen your body to cope with the increasing weight of the pregnancy, and the birth.' If only mainstream health would adopt the same approach.

In the early days of January 2016 my husband takes us away for a child-free break in the countryside. We walk through muddy forest together, climb over stiles – him marvelling that despite being heavily pregnant I can still swing a leg over with ease – and laugh, breathless, climbing the hills. In an outdoor heated pool, I decide to take the plunge. I look up at the January skies, the leaves on the trees, and breathe, exhilarated. I have done this before, in London, with friends, at a time in my life when exercise came more easily. We swam all year round, but it was always most special in winter, when others did not dare, when we had the pool to ourselves, just the hardcore swimmers – many of them older than us – with some crows and bare branches overhead for company. One magical Christmas Eve we swam in the snow. Years later, here I am, swimming in deepest winter again. It feels as amazing now as it did then. Just one little swim. One little run. One little walk. That's all it takes, and you're right back there. You haven't got lost. It hasn't gone away. It's all there just waiting for you, whenever you're ready to grab it.

Acknowledgements

Since my husband and I first got together, he has always encouraged me to write a book. A decade on and it's finally happened. Thank you, Leon – *so much* – for helping me get so far: engaging in endless conversations about women and sport, looking after our daughter, providing pep talks and even paying my rent when I couldn't afford to. The practical support has been amazing, but that you actually liked the book, and believed in it, made me smile to the rooftops. I love you.

Thank you to my daughter Ella for being brilliant, so accepting of 'mummy writing a book'. You inspire me every single day, and it's a privilege to watch you grow up and tackle the world with such aplomb. I love you very much, and I am very proud to be your mum.

A huge thank you to my mum and dad, who arrived in this country many decades ago with no connection to this place, and yet have ended up rooted here by children, grandchildren, and now a real-life published book. Thank you for your love, interest, ideas, conversations and support. And for seeing beyond the sport, and what else it signifies. Thank you to my big brother Stef, for ensuring that I never supported Tottenham; I miss you every day. And thank you to Frankie for an education in the

Chicago Bears, a shared love of athletics, and showing us all that sport is great at any time in life (even downhill skiing in your eighties).

An enormous thank you to everyone who has helped look after Ella when I needed to write – mostly my parents, parents-in-law, and my daughter's nursery teachers. Childcare is a soulless word, but you've all proved that spending time with a small person isn't about shuffling a parcel around, it's about creating relationships and having fun. I never had to worry or feel guilty about leaving my daughter to write. As a working mum I realize just how privileged a position that is to be in.

Thank you to my amazing friends who, mostly, are not sports fans but gave me all their enthusiasm, ideas and feedback anyway, along with cheerleader levels of support. Tamzin Davis, all those cups of tea and chats meant so much, thank you for being such a loyal and supportive friend. Thank you Clare O'Driscoll, Sophie Loi-Shaw and Dr Lucy Irving for the love, and Arsenal memories; Elaine Moore and Madeleine Bretting-ham for brilliant writer's insights, constructive criticism and running in mud, you amazing women! Sophie Maqsood, Emmi Poteliakhoff, Martha Davis, Anjana Gadgil, Amy Lawrence, Amy Pollard and Kate Streeter, for allowing me to so freely pick their brains about exercise and motherhood. And to my sister-in-law Natasha Mann, who was so generous with her support (and very nearly hooked me up with Mary J. Blige. OMG. All hail!).

To the wonderful Women in Football board members, past and present, who encouraged me to find my own voice long before this book came into being. And to the many women and men in the sports industry who took time out of their schedules to be interviewed, or helped direct me to great interviewees – I am so grateful to you. Thank you, in particular, Jacqui Oatley, Shelley Alexander, Judy Murray, Kelly Sotherton, Marilyn Okoro, Joanna Manning-Cooper, Sue Mott, Jo Bostock, Christine Bowmaker, Michelle Moore, Kate Bosomworth and Simone Harvey and the boxing mums. And thank you Mark Barden for being so understanding when I needed time off work.

Thank you to those who set me on my sports writing journey – the inimitable Gaffer, Eggy and the old *Observer* sports desk, everyone at *Guardian* and *Observer* sport who have supported my career since and/or my sabbatical to write this book, and Don McRae who has always been so generous with his time and advice. It was Don who led me to Curtis Brown and my lovely agent Richard Pike, who in turn led me to Robin Harvie, Laura Langlois and all the other great people at Macmillan. Thank you all so much for turning an impossible concept of a book into a reality, not batting an eyelid when I became pregnant and – best of all – making the writing such an enjoyable experience along the way.

Finally, to all women and girls everywhere, from centuries past, and in years to come, who all just want to bust out a move. I salute you.

Permissions Acknowledgements

Notes

1   Allison Glock, 'The Conversation with Actor/Writer/Director/Producer (And Runner) Lena Dunham,' ESPNW, 21 September 2015.

2   Anna Kessel, 'Martina Navratilova battles the test of time', *Observer*, 4 July 2010.

3   Anna Kessel, 'Mel C: I'm scared of the bike. You can really hurt yourself if you fall off', Small Talk, *Guardian*, 9 May 2014.

4   Claudia Rankine, 'The Meaning of Serena Williams', *New York Times Magazine*, 25 August 2015.

5   Dave Zirin, 'Serena Williams is Today's Muhammad Ali', *The Nation*, 14 July 2015.

6   Anna Kessel, 'The Star Next Door', *Observer Sport Monthly*, 23 November 2008.

7   Naomi Alderman, 'There's No Morality in Exercise: I'm a Fat Person and Made a Successful Fitness App', medium.com, 11 February 2015.

8   Juliet Macur, 'Fighting for the Body She Was Born With', *New York Times*, 6 October 2014.

9   Roberta 'Bobbi' Gibb, 'A Run Of One's Own', runningpast. com.

10 John Cunningham, 'Avon Calling As 200 Runners Join Women-Only Marathon', *Guardian*, 1 August 1980.

11 Anna Kessel, 'Liz McColgan-Nuttall is Introducing Girls in Qatar to the Joys of Running', *Observer*, 21 December 2014.

12 Anna Kessel, 'Olympic gold and unbeaten rowing success a close thing for Helen Glover,' *Observer*, 16 November 2014.

13 George Parker, 'Power Games', *Financial Times Magazine*, 7 March 2008.

14 Anna Kessel, 'Goalball – the Silent Sport Changing Visually Impaired Women's Lives', *Guardian*, 28 August 2014.

15 Mark Hodgkinson, 'Wimbledon 2009: Jelena Jankovic Suffers Dizziness in Defeat by Melanie Oudin', *Telegraph*, 27 June 2009.

16 'Serena Says She's Suffered From Migraines for Years', ESPN.com, Associated Press, 11 April 2005.

17 Kiran Gandhi, 'Sisterhood, Blood and Boobs at the London Marathon 2015,' kirangandhi.com, 26 April 2015.

18 Joe Fassler, 'How Doctors Take Women's Pain Less Seriously', the *Atlantic*, 15 October 2015.

19 Anna Kessel, 'The Bedroom Olympics', *Observer Sport Monthly*, 3 February 2008.

20 Ronda Rousey TV interview with Jim Rome, *Showtime*, 29 November 2012.

21 Suzi Godson, 'He can't keep up with me in bed', Body and Soul section in the *Sunday Times Magazine*, 17 October 2015, p. 8.

22 Jennifer Quinn, 'The Myths of Sex Before Sport', *BBC Online News Magazine*, 12 August 2004.

23 Emma Bridgewater, *Toast & Marmalade: Stories from the Kitchen Dresser, A Memoir*. Saltyard Books, 2014.

24 Anna Kessel, 'Emma Croker: England's Mother of Multi-Taskers', *Observer*, 28 October 2012.

25 Anna Kessel, 'Jill Ellis Feels At Home Plotting Path To World Cup Glory For USA Big Names', *Guardian*, 8 June 2015.

26 Afua Hirsch, 'The Mothers of Africa', *Guardian*, 20 July 2012.

27 Ranjana Srivastava, '"What's a Uterus?" Health Illiteracy Could be the Death of Us', *Guardian*, 8 September 2015.

28 Anna Tyzack, 'How Laura Trott Became the Face of the Women's Institute', *Telegraph*, 26 July 2015.

29 Nick Hornby, *Fever Pitch*, Gollancz, 1992.

30 'Delia Smith interview', BBC Radio Norfolk, reproduced on BBC online, 2 March 2005, www.bbc.co.uk/norfolk/content/articles/2005/03/02/sport_delia_smith_inter-view_20050302_feature.shtml

31 Lee Hurley, 'You Won't Believe the Sexist Abuse STILL Aimed at Female Football Fans. I Do Because I Used To Be A Woman', *Mirror*, 3 April 2014.

32 Anna Kessel, 'Gascoigne Off To A Winning Start', *Observer*, 30 October 2005.

33 Cameron Carter, 'A Female Commentator on the BBC', *When Saturday Comes*, Issue 244, June 2007.

34 Katie Nolan, 'Why Boycotting the NFL Because of Ray Rice is not the Answer', YouTube, 9 September 2014, https://www.youtube.com/watch?v=HaHIzIXrS0w

35 Richard Deitsch, 'CBS Sports Network to Debut Weekly All-Female Sports Talk Show', *Sports Illustrated*, 30 September 2014.

36 Anna Kessel, 'Paid To Play: Levelling the Field for Women's Professional Sport', *Observer*, 31 May 2015.

37 Anna Kessel, 'Reanne Evans Aims to Bridge Gender Gap at World Snooker Championship', *Guardian*, 5 March 2015.